T0187054

Unheard

The Medical Practice of Silencing

Unheard

The Medical Practice of Silencing

Dr Rageshri Dhairyawan

TRAPEZE

First published in Great Britain in 2024 by Trapeze,
an imprint of The Orion Publishing Group Ltd
Carmelite House, 50 Victoria Embankment
London EC4Y 0CZ

An Hachette UK Company

1 3 5 7 9 10 8 6 4 2

Extract on p.226: Lines from 'The Unsung' by Hanan Issa,
reproduced with permission from the poet.

A CIP catalogue record for this book is
available from the British Library.

ISBN (Hardback) 978 1 3987 1869 2
ISBN (eBook) 978 1 3987 1871 5
ISBN (Audio) 978 1 3987 1872 2

Typeset at The Spartan Press Ltd,
Lymington, Hants

Printed and bound in Great Britain by Clays Ltd,
Elcograf S.p.A.

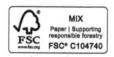

www.orionbooks.co.uk

For those who are striving to be heard

Contents

Introduction

Failing to Listen

I know what it feels like to not be heard as a patient. Not being heard or being taken seriously in healthcare seems to be an almost universal experience. At least that's how it seems from my perspective, as a doctor, researcher and patient. Most people I've spoken to have a story about how it happened to them, or to someone they know. It may have happened to you. We often talk about delivering health*care*, but for far too many people it doesn't feel like healthcare services *care about them*. This is a book about who gets listened to and who doesn't in medicine and how this leads to a culture of silencing that exacerbates health inequities, unjust differences in health, on an individual and global scale. It's also about what we can do to make sure everyone's voice is equally heard and valued; a prescription to close the gap for the most marginalised in society and by doing this, improving healthcare for all.

In 2013, I was admitted to hospital with excruciating abdominal pain. I was in the middle of my third cycle of in vitro fertilisation (IVF) treatment and had just had eggs collected from my ovaries the day before. The pain had started slowly, but by that evening I was lying on the bathroom floor at home, trying to find relief from the cold tiles. I felt as if a heavy metal shovel was scraping away at the lining of my abdomen. My usual painkillers had barely scratched the surface and I was in agony. Pain was an old adversary of mine. I had been diagnosed with endometriosis, a menstrual condition for which pain is a characteristic feature, several years earlier, but this felt different and very wrong. I was worried I had developed ovarian torsion, a complication of IVF, where an ovary so swollen from hormonal stimulation can twist on its stalk. This cuts off its blood supply, starving it of oxygen, causing severe pain. If not untwisted by a surgeon, the ovary dies. My husband came home to find me writhing on the floor in distress. He quickly took me to hospital where the emergency department team gave me strong analgesia and admitted me to the gynaecology ward for further investigation. At the time, the pain was traumatic enough but I didn't realise the real ordeal was still to come.

The next day an internal scan ruled out ovarian torsion, and my medical team attributed my symptoms to 'just' a flare up of endometriosis from the IVF hormones. Without the more 'serious' diagnosis of ovarian torsion, which would have required urgent surgery, for the rest of my admission I was made to feel like a fraud for still complaining of pain. On the ward, I kept having to plead for more pain relief, but I was repeatedly dismissed, my concerns minimised by the healthcare team. Despite at this point being a senior doctor in the NHS, a consultant with almost ten years' experience of treating patients and leading teams, I wasn't able to speak up for myself. I felt humiliated. It was only through my husband's advocacy, talking to the healthcare team again and again, that I got the pain medication I needed and was discharged after three days.

More than ten years later, I can still remember how scared and helpless I felt. I had no faith that the team responsible for my care would look after me. I had been treated as though I was an unreliable narrator, an attention seeker, someone trying to get strong opioids through dishonest means. It was not the care I expected or deserved. Unsurprisingly, the IVF cycle failed – the embryos they transferred during the admission did not make themselves at home in my stressed out, frightened body. Another precious chance to be a mother gone.

I didn't complain at the time, because I didn't want to be seen as more of a nuisance. But I came to regret this and blamed myself for not speaking up, for not standing up for myself. Although the physical recovery was quick, the feelings of shame lingered. I was ashamed because I felt as if I had been silenced by the system designed to protect me, both during the admission and afterwards.

I was worried that my care would suffer further if I appeared to the healthcare team to be 'making a fuss'. I didn't want to be *that* patient, the problem admission who elicited eye rolls and complaints from ward staff for wasting their valuable time.

I also felt responsible for other women after me who might end up in my situation. By not speaking up, was I part of the problem? What might happen to less informed patients in my situation? To those who couldn't speak English? And what if my condition had been more serious, even life-threatening – would I have made it out of hospital? I was fortunate to have my husband support me, but not everyone is lucky enough to have someone to advocate for them. This contributed to a sense of guilt which stayed with me long afterwards.

In 2022, renowned African American tennis player, Serena Williams wrote in *Elle* about her own experience of not being heard in healthcare.[1] After giving birth to her daughter Olympia in 2018, she suffered life-threatening complications. The day after an emergency caesarean section, she started to feel short of breath. She had been treated for a serious blood clot in her lungs in the past and having recently come off blood thinning medication for an operation, she was worried she may have another. When she reported her concerns to her nurse she was told, 'I think all of this medicine is making you talk crazy.' Thankfully Serena was able to persuade her medical team to take her worries seriously. As she suspected, a scan showed several blood clots in her lungs and she received the life-saving treatment she needed.

She says of the experience, 'Giving birth to my baby, it turned out, was a test for how loud and how often I would have to call out before I was finally heard. No one was really listening to what I was saying.'

I think this experience of not being heard may be one of two things I can claim to have in common with Serena Williams, who I consider to be one of the greatest athletes the world has ever seen. I have never excelled at sport (I don't think brief spells on the school netball and hockey teams count) and to my knowledge, she doesn't have a medical degree. What we have in common is that we were both not taken seriously in situations where we were at our most vulnerable. The second thing is that we are both women of colour. Women of colour and especially Black women widely report being unheard, dismissed and disbelieved in healthcare. And this leads to real and avoidable harm. This has been particularly highlighted in recent reports of maternal deaths in the United States and the United Kingdom. Black women in the US are three times more likely than white women to die in pregnancy. In the UK, they are four times more likely and other women of colour two times more likely to die. A consistent theme in investigations is that these women and their relatives were not listened to, or taken seriously by healthcare staff when they felt something was wrong.[2-5] In Brazil, a national study found racial disparities in care during pregnancy and childbirth, which showed a gradient based on skin colour – Black women experienced the worst care, followed by brown women, with white women experiencing the best care.[6] These disparities are also seen for their babies – in the UK, Black babies are twice as likely to be stillborn or die within twenty-eight days of birth than white babies, while Asian babies are one and a half times as likely.[7] When interviewed about their experiences of healthcare in pregnancy, many bereaved parents talked about being stereotyped by healthcare staff – for Black women, being characterised as 'feisty' or 'dramatic' when in pain or afraid; for Asian women being dismissed as having health anxiety. Over half felt that their care was worse or different due to their ethnicity.[8]

Differences in the treatment of pain have also been widely reported. A large review looking back at twenty years of pain management in the US shows that African Americans are less likely to receive adequate pain relief and that this is a significant safety issue.[9] This has been found to be due to stereotypes used by healthcare staff that Black people are 'drug-addicts', and false biological beliefs about their bodies being better able to tolerate pain.[10] Historically women have had their pain dismissed – there is a wealth of evidence from several countries showing women suffer delays in getting pain relief and often are not given enough.[11-13]

Despite being Serena Williams, one of the greatest athletes the

4

world has ever seen, she is also a Black woman in a healthcare system where racist and sexist biases are historically ingrained, and this overrode her fame. If this could happen to Serena Williams or to me, a senior doctor, it can happen to anyone, but particularly women and people from minoritised communities. As Williams later wrote, 'Being heard and appropriately treated was the difference between life and death for me; I know those statistics would be different if the medical establishment listened to every Black woman's experience.'[14]

How can we get to a place where the medical establishment listens to every Black woman's experience? And to others who are routinely not heard or believed?

This is what I will explore in this book. I've worked as a doctor in some of the most economically and socially unequal areas in England over the last twenty years and seen first-hand the devastating impacts of health inequalities on individual patients. Their stories have stayed with me, but their voices are also those least likely to be heard in public conversations about healthcare. As Indian writer Arundhati Roy said, they are not 'voiceless', but 'the deliberately silenced, or the preferably unheard.'[15] They are not being heard by their doctors, by researchers or by policymakers. Their health needs are not being prioritised, and they are underserved by the very institutions that should be working for them.

As a doctor, I'm also guilty of not always listening to the best of my ability – this has never been intentional but is something I've reflected on a lot. It's often been at times when I've felt unable to listen, because I've been rushed or tired such as during a busy night shift or at the end of an overbooked clinic. Or when I've felt uncomfortable listening, because what I've heard is distressing and I can't provide a quick fix by writing a prescription. Like most of my colleagues, I came into the profession to help people feel better; to provide empathy and high-quality care. I would like to work in a system where I feel better trained to listen and have the capacity to do so.

The need to address disparities in health has become increasingly urgent. Their widespread nature has been uncovered by the

COVID-19 pandemic and they are predicted to worsen over the next few years, due to rises in the cost of living and continuing austerity policies. Health inequities are defined as unfair and avoidable systemic differences in health between groups. They are a form of injustice.[16] They have existed in most areas of health for a long time. For example, in my speciality of sexual health, high rates of gonorrhoea in the UK were first reported among Black Caribbean men in the 1950s.[17] More than seventy years on, this continues to be the case with annual statistics showing similar findings, exposing ineffective strategies and perhaps even insufficient will to effectively resolve this inequity.[18]

Highlighting and addressing health inequality has been a guiding force in my career, through my clinical practice and policy work, my advocacy with patient groups and my research. This empowers me to speak up and is the reason I'm writing this book. For example, through research, I've produced evidence to show how the health inequities I've seen in real life experienced by individual patients are not one-offs but play out at a broader population level. This means they might get more attention from policymakers, a step towards getting the resources to start reversing them. One instance was when I started to notice that many of the people I was treating with advanced HIV disease were Black or from other racially minoritised groups. I wanted to see if this was a trend or something unique to our centre. I approached other researchers and we found that this was happening nationally – there were differences in HIV treatment outcomes by ethnic group.[19] Racially minoritised people with HIV are more likely to be diagnosed at an advanced stage of illness and less likely to be consistently on effective treatment, increasing their risk of illness and death. This is probably due to social and economic difficulties accessing healthcare services, but may also reflect poor experiences of healthcare and mistrust in staff. This finding has been taken up by national HIV policymakers with plans made to tackle it.[20]

There are many causes of health inequities, but most are due to what are termed 'the social determinants of health', the conditions in which we are born, grow, work, live and age, and wider systems such as economic policies and societal norms. In the UK, health equity expert Professor Sir Michael Marmot showed in his landmark report, 'Health Equity in England: The Marmot Review 10 Years On', that between 2010 and 2020, life expectancy had decreased for the poorest 10 per cent of women in England, due to policies of austerity.[21] Being poor is one of the main risk factors for ill health and early death. While unequal social and economic conditions are the most important cause of poor health, healthcare *itself* can cause inequities to worsen, rather than alleviating them. People's experiences of healthcare differ widely and can be dependent on aspects of their identity – their gender, age, ethnicity, class, religion, ability and sexual orientation. Put simply, healthcare is less safe for some people than others. This is a huge injustice.

For example, people of colour are more likely to experience discrimination, inappropriate restraint, inadequate pain relief and medication errors.[22] Many of these harms are due to poor communication between healthcare staff and patients. In the UK, 23 per cent of LGBTQ+ patients, rising to 40 per cent in transgender patients, have experienced discrimination from healthcare workers. One in five LGBTQ+ people have reported they avoid accessing healthcare due to fear of this.[23] Trans and non-binary people were also less likely to be involved in decisions about their care when seeing a GP (general practitioner).[24] A global review found that due to ageism, older people were less likely to receive certain treatments.[25] People with a learning disability in the UK have a much lower life expectancy than the general population and this differs by ethnic background.[26] Those from a racially minoritised community can expect to live just thirty-four years on average and those who are white, sixty-two years. The groups that suffer most patient safety incidents are also those that report that they are not listened to or taken seriously by healthcare professionals.[27] These poor experiences of care have a lasting impact on trust – communities who have suffered harm due to prejudice are more likely to mistrust healthcare staff and institutions. This was seen clearly with the lower uptake of the COVID-19 vaccination by some racially minoritised groups in the UK.[28]

In a speech at the Convention of the Medical Committee for Human Rights held in Chicago in 1966, Martin Luther King Jr. said, 'Of all the forms of inequality, injustice in health care is the most shocking and inhumane.'[29] People are at their most vulnerable when unwell, and healthcare is meant to ease their suffering, not make it worse. We should all feel safe and respected in these situations and fundamental to this is feeling heard and believed. Not being listened to in a medical situation is a significant cause of illness and death that needs to be addressed and so far, little progress has been made. As a solution, patients are often told to speak up, to be louder and advocate for themselves better. But perhaps this is a form of victim-blaming? Why should the responsibility to speak up lie with those not listened to, rather than the healthcare system whose job it is to listen carefully? And for some patient groups this may even be dangerous – they may get punished for asserting themselves, particularly those that may be incorrectly stereotyped as being inherently more aggressive, like Black women.

My experience of not being heard as a patient has profoundly changed how I view patient care. I'm a more careful listener now, and I take a patient's pain very seriously. But I don't think it should take the experience of being a patient to make doctors better listeners. I think this is a skill that can be taught and encouraged through changing how healthcare systems operate and how we train doctors and other professionals. Through research and reading, I've learnt of ways in which we can make this happen.

*

With this book, I bring a new perspective to the conversation on addressing health inequity, arguing that better listening is needed throughout healthcare and research to close the health gap for minoritised people. Through understanding how it feels to be on either side of the consultation, both the side with more power and the side with less, I have seen in so many cases how listening can bring more equality to our encounters. Undoubtedly, the first step to listening better is awareness of how marginalised voices are silenced in many areas of healthcare and research, and how this exacerbates differences in health outcomes. I'll be detailing the fascinating and shocking stories and histories that show us clearly what needs to change, so that we can see and understand *why* listening is so important before I describe exactly *how* we can do better.

At the centre of this narrative are the patients. I want to use my power and expertise as a doctor to facilitate their voices, because it is often deemed that only doctors' opinions matter. I'll be asking why patients are not heard in healthcare and how are they silenced. Why do some individuals or groups get listened to less than others? And how is this linked to societal bias? I'll be weaving in real-life stories from patients, as well as some doctors and researchers, whose voices have been historically less heard and urgently need to be considered. I want this book to feel like an empowering tool that anyone can use at any stage of their life to better advocate for themselves in healthcare, and so I will be including resources and advice at the end of each chapter so you can take the learnings here out into the real world.

An important part of this book is that I am a doctor, with extensive experience and knowledge of healthcare, and perhaps that is why you picked up this book in the first place. I'll be reflecting on my own experiences of not listening as a doctor and investigating what gets in the way of doctors listening. I will illustrate how this starts at medical school where we learn to doubt what our patients say and develop a sense of hubris. This is also where we are taught the language of medicine, which has scepticism of patient testimonies ingrained within it. I'll explore how true listening can be uncomfortable for doctors, making us put up boundaries and even question what our role is. Doctors also don't listen to each other and this can have profound effects on patient care directly and indirectly. When this happens to minoritised doctors, they are made to feel like 'outsiders' and this can lead to impostor syndrome, burnout and their departure from the healthcare workforce. I'll also show how when minoritised doctors and researchers are silenced, this causes gaps in medical knowledge, which impacts patients. *Who* gets to do research and produce knowledge is dependent on enduring power hierarchies in global health, which have historically operated since colonialism. Looking back to the roots of Western medicine, you can see why certain kinds of knowledge have been traditionally prized in medicine, while others are neglected. This includes knowledge produced by patients which has been systematically devalued.

To preserve anonymity, the patient stories I present are not specific individual patients. They are an amalgamation of patients I have seen over the years, or patient testimonies I've heard in interviews or published reports. My hope is that they bring the issues I discuss to life for the reader. Likewise, the doctor and researcher stories are fictionalised, but based on first- or second-hand accounts. I live and work in the UK, so this book will be mostly written with this perspective and that of Western healthcare systems. I appreciate therefore that while many of these issues are universal, not every element will apply in every country. However, I hope that the insights I provide will benefit doctors, researchers and patients everywhere. Also, while I'll be talking about any healthcare professional not listening, which includes doctors, nurses, allied health professionals among others, for simplicity I will mostly be referring to doctors and researchers.

It is important we recognise these issues; if healthcare is ever to improve, it must learn from its failings, and we must accept it is as flawed as the people who have built it. However, there are always positives and progress, and so I will be speaking to people who are leading this change, demonstrating that there are ways – practical, realistic and achievable ways – in which people from minoritised groups can be heard.

The British philosopher Miranda Fricker wrote that 'Being understood, expressing oneself, being able to contribute to meaning-making are basic human capabilities and constitutive of a dignified life.'[30] Being heard is an integral part of what makes us human. Listening and expressing empathy is one of our most basic yet fundamental methods of connecting. Going back to these basics is a real way for us to progress and by doing so, I believe we could have a healthcare system that no longer dehumanises the most marginalised, but listens to them, so that no one goes unheard.

I

Dismissed

How Patients Are Silenced

It's Michael's fourth day in hospital, and he's not feeling any better. His legs are hurting, he's weak, and his appetite has deserted him. He's been unable to sleep as the patient in the bed next to him had been coughing all night, and by the time he finally dropped off, he was woken to have his vital signs measured. After checking his blood pressure, heart rate, oxygen levels and temperature, the healthcare assistant told him, 'You're tachycardic.' *Hardly surprising*, he thought. His heart was racing at over 100 beats per minute because he was in constant pain.

He'd been admitted with another sickle cell crisis, his third this year. He's had sickle cell disease as long as he can remember. His mum told him he was tested as a baby because it ran in the family. Sickle cell, he'd been taught, was a genetic condition that affected the shape of the red cells in his blood, turning them into the shape of a sickle, a 'C'. This made them sticky. He was first admitted to hospital with a sickle cell crisis when he was ten – he can remember the doctors on the ward trying to explain that the sickle cells had stuck together, blocking the small blood vessels to a part of his body, starving it of oxygen.

Now aged twenty-eight, he still dreaded having a crisis as they were extremely painful and often lasted up to a week. This meant taking time off work, a job he was growing to love as a teacher in a primary school. It was sometimes hard going, but he had started to feel like he was making a difference to the children he taught.

This week it was his class's turn to lead assembly, a presentation on the renowned British-Jamaican nurse Mary Seacole. They'd practised all last week, and now he was going to miss seeing them perform. His colleagues said they'd send him a video, but it wasn't the same as being there. He was exhausted and fed up.

'So, Michael, tell me, what's your pain score? How would you rate your pain on a scale from one to ten with ten being the worst pain you can imagine?' asks Sarah, the ward nurse on her evening drug round.

'It's ten...' replies Michael quietly, his teeth gritted. He's not sure a number can fully describe how he's currently feeling. 'Like I'm being tortured' would be a better description, along with 'terrified'.

'Ten?' Sarah exclaims. 'You don't look as bad as a ten. Are you sure?'

She thinks to herself, *If it was really a ten, surely he'd be crying and screaming. He must be exaggerating. Here he is, in hospital again, always asking for more pain relief. More morphine. That's why he's here. He's looking for more drugs. He gets more and more difficult every time he comes in. I'm fed up with looking after him.*

She sighs and says, 'Look, Michael, I'm sorry you're in so much pain, but it's only been an hour since we last gave you something. I can't give you more than paracetamol. You'll just have to wait.' She pushes the drug trolley forward and continues her round of the patients in the bay.

An hour later, Michael presses the buzzer by his bed. She finishes her task, washes her hands, taking deep breaths to prepare herself, and walks over to him.

As Sarah approaches, she sees that he is now sitting upright in the bed, muscles rigid with tension, hospital gown and sheets damp with sweat. He cries out, 'Please! Can you help me? I'm in agony. Surely I'm due for some more painkillers now.'

'I'm not sure... I'll speak to my supervisor and see what he says,' she replies. At the nursing station she spots Mark, the nurse in charge. She sighs with relief, thinking, *Mark always knows what to do with demanding patients – he'll be able to help.*

Sarah explains the situation to him. Mark rolls his eyes and replies,

'Hmm... surely it can't be that bad. But if it really is a ten, I guess we'd better talk to the on-call doctor. Can you contact them?'

After several attempts, Sarah gets hold of the doctor who apologises for not answering the call sooner – she's been at a cardiac arrest on a neighbouring ward. 'What can I do to help?' she asks.

Sarah replies, 'Thank you for answering, Dr Singh. Mark suggested I call you – it's that patient Michael, you know, the one with the sickle cell – he's been admitted again. He's being a bit difficult – I gave him some Oramorph just two hours ago, but he says he's still in pain – says its ten out of ten. Honestly, I don't know how it can be. I do wonder if he's exaggerating... but that's what he says. What shall I do? Can I give him some more, or maybe something else?'

Dr Singh replies, 'Oh, I remember him... I was on call the last time he was in and something similar happened then – he took ages and a lot of morphine to settle! OK, give him half a dose and keep an eye on him. If it's still bad, give me a call. I need to go and see a patient with chest pain on the cardiology ward – they sound really unwell. It doesn't sound like I need to come up and see the sickle cell?'

Sarah agrees. 'No, I don't think you need to come up here. It's not urgent. Thanks doctor.' She smiles to herself, satisfied they have a plan, and goes to the drug room.

'Here you go, Michael. I've spoken to the on-call doctor. Here's some more Oramorph,' Sarah says, measuring out the clear liquid into a paper cup.

'Thank you... but is that it? Not even an injection...? That won't do much.' Michael is now distraught. 'When am I going to see a doctor? In fact, when am I going to see the sickle cell team? I've been asking for them every day since I came into hospital. It's been four days now and I still haven't seen my specialist. What's going on?'

During a sickle cell crisis, national guidelines recommend that patients are seen by haematologists (blood specialists) when they are admitted to hospital. Patients should be given oxygen, pain relief and intravenous fluids, but sometimes blood transfusions and other specific drugs are needed, which specialists are trained to advise on.

Sarah replies sternly, 'This is what the on-call doctor has instructed me to do. When your doctors do the ward round tomorrow morning, ask them about the sickle cell team then.'

She's annoyed, thinking, *It's not my fault they haven't been to see him. I'm not sure the ward doctors have even contacted them. Why should they? These sickle cell patients don't need anything special – just a drip, some oxygen and some painkillers. It's not more complicated than that – they just think they're special. Once they've been in for a few days and had enough, they miss their home comforts and discharge themselves.*

She locks the drug room, thinking about her upcoming break – it's been a busy evening, they've been understaffed and on top of that she's had to deal with Michael being a nuisance. It cannot come soon enough.

Michael is lying cocooned in his bed sheets, his head covered, weeping softly. He can feel the morphine starting to take effect and his breaths start to deepen. He cautiously starts to unfurl his aching limbs and settles into the mattress, now soaking with his sweat.

He thinks, *Each time I come in here, it gets harder. Why do I have to shout and beg for my medication? It's not my fault. I didn't choose to be born with sickle cell... at least when I was a child, they felt sorry for me. I even used to get treats from the nurses – sweets and chocolates. Those were the days... Now, every time they speak to me, I can tell they're thinking 'he's a liar'. Even when they don't speak to me, I can tell they're thinking it. It's the way they tut, they roll their eyes, they look down on me. The way they speak about me when they think I can't hear them. If only they could understand what it's like to live with this illness. Where's the empathy? It makes me not want to come to hospital, even if I'm really sick. I'm only here because I can't cope at home.*

*

Michael's experience is sadly one that people with sickle cell suffer far too commonly. Sickle cell disease is an invisible condition – you can't tell someone has it just from looking at them. Due to this, its gravity often goes unrecognised by healthcare staff who can view people with sickle cell disease as a nuisance, or even as drug addicts exaggerating their symptoms. The diagnosis carries significant stigma, which can make it even harder for patients to speak up.

This is despite sickle cell disease being the most common genetic disorder in the world and a serious condition that can affect the whole body in different ways. As well as causing crises, the sickle cells die more quickly than normal red blood cells, causing anaemia and constant fatigue. Long-term complications can include blindness, strokes, heart attacks, chronic pain and infections. Patients need to be looked after from birth throughout their life by a specialist team of doctors and nurses. This makes them particularly in need of a healthcare team that they can trust and work with. While sickle cell patients often speak highly of their specialist teams, they report very different experiences of care when being looked after by non-specialists.

Wellness coach, author and speaker Cheryl Telfer has written about living with the condition, saying, 'Even when you're not in crisis, it's a disease that never leaves your side.' She describes the pain as being 'soul-crushing' and the inadequate response of healthcare professionals: 'The sad truth is that many sicklers feel unheard, and many times gaslit.'[1]

Research shows that the negative attitudes they encounter in healthcare settings are often 'underpinned by racism'.[2] Sickle cell disease is an inherited condition common among people with heritage in North Africa, South Asia, the Middle East and the Southern Mediterranean. These are areas where malaria is rife and the abnormal sickle cells can be protective. In the UK and US, due to migration patterns and colonialism, people with sickle cell disease are often of Black ethnicity. There is a common misconception that it only affects Black people.

This combination of stigma around the diagnosis itself and racism means that sickle cell patients have historically suffered poor care, and many have even died due to neglect in hospital. Tragically, people with sickle cell disease are still dying in hospitals – these are avoidable deaths and a catastrophic failure of care.

Tyrone Airey, a popular singer known by his recording name Tai Malone, died at the age of forty-six years in a London hospital in March 2021 from a morphine overdose.[3] He had been admitted with a sickle cell crisis. He'd first had a crisis when he was four years old, and as an adult was getting them three to four times a year. When the chest and back pain got too excruciating for him to cope with, he'd seek hospital care. On this occasion, he was given a pump which allows patients to press a button for more morphine when they need it, putting them in control of their pain relief, but within safe limits. However, the inquest into his death found that the nursing staff did not have enough training to manage or monitor the use of the pump. Signs that he was getting too much morphine were missed. Local and national guidance on the care of sickle cell patients was not followed. The coroner ruled that neglect contributed to Tyrone's death.[4]

Evan Nathan Smith also died in a London hospital aged just twenty-one in April 2019, from the complications of sickle cell disease and a failure of care.[5] A day before his admission, he had a routine procedure carried out on his gallbladder. At home, he developed a high temperature, dehydration and a yellowing of his eyes due to jaundice. After being assessed at the hospital, he was moved to a general ward. However, there was no bed for him there and he was placed on a trolley in the corridor of the ward temporarily. The trolley did not have a patient buzzer which allows patients to call the nurse for help. Over the next few days, Evan became increasingly unwell with worsening fevers and jaundice, breathlessness and joint pain. The medical team felt that he was likely to have an infection due to his gallbladder procedure. He was treated with antibiotics with the plan to have another surgical procedure to wash out anything causing the infection.

It was not until five days after his admission that Evan was seen by a haematologist, a blood specialist who provides care for people with sickle cell disease. In that time, he had told his father that he had asked the nurses for more oxygen but had been refused it. Heartbreakingly, he felt so desperate that he rang 999 to ask for oxygen. He was told they couldn't help because he was already in hospital where oxygen was available. Despite this, he couldn't access it because the healthcare staff had denied it to him. The haematologist recognised that Evan was experiencing a sickle cell crisis and arranged for treatment with oxygen and an exchange transfusion, which replaces the patient's abnormally sickled blood with normal blood. Sadly, this proved to be too late. Evan's condition got worse, and despite being moved to the intensive-care unit he died one week after he had been admitted.

An inquest into his death was instigated by Evan's parents, to find answers to why their son had died in hospital so unexpectedly. The coroner, Dr Andrew Walker, reported that Evan's death had been avoidable – 'The delay in treating Mr Smith with a timely exchange transfusion was the cause of his death.'[6] He found a lack of awareness of sickle cell disease among the healthcare team, which meant that they were preoccupied with the alternative diagnosis of an infection following his gallbladder procedure. The coroner pointed out that as per national guidance, he should have been flagged up to the specialist haematology team when admitted so they could see him much sooner. The inquest into Evan's death led to an inquiry into avoidable deaths and failures of care for sickle cell patients in hospitals in the UK. This was carried out by the All-Party Parliamentary Group (APPG) on Sickle Cell and Thalassaemia and the Sickle Cell Society charity. Aptly named 'No One's Listening', the report was published in November 2021.[7]

'No One's Listening' found evidence that the poor care experienced by Tyrone and Evan was widespread among sickle cell patients admitted to general wards and emergency departments. National care standards were rarely followed and there was low awareness of sickle cell disease among healthcare professionals, and inadequate training and investment in care. Finally, it described frequent reports of negative attitudes towards patients with sickle cell, which were reinforced by racism.[8]

It's very hard to hear of such deaths still occurring. The accounts remind me of how I felt being denied pain relief when admitted with the complications of endometriosis, which like sickle cell disease is an invisible condition. Only, I knew that my illness wasn't life-threatening. I can't imagine how scary it would have felt to know I may die from medical neglect. As a doctor, while I know that avoidable deaths happen, it is still shocking to hear individual accounts of patients with sickle cell and to see how common the negative attitudes, stigma and racism they experience are. For me, this shows why a change in culture to one that prioritises listening is so important and urgent. It will save lives. This drives me to be part of this change.

These preventable deaths happened despite decades of tireless work from pioneering sickle cell disease healthcare workers and community advocates. They collectively fought for the acknowledgement of the condition from policymakers, for screening and specialist care. In the UK, these include Dame Professor Elizabeth Anionwu, the first specialist sickle cell nurse, Dr Neville Clare, who launched the Organisation for Sickle Cell Anaemia Research in 1976, and the Sickle Cell Society. In the US, one of the pioneers was Dr Charles F. Whitten, founder of the Sickle Cell Disease Association of America. It's no coincidence that many of the pioneers in sickle cell disease advocacy come from Black communities. Minoritised healthcare professionals often advocate for diseases that affect their communities. This highlights the importance of these healthcare professionals and researchers themselves being heard by their peers.

This advocacy needs to continue. Sickle cell disease affects millions of people around the world, particularly those that live in poorer countries. It has been underfunded and neglected by researchers until recently. There have also been international calls from doctors, researchers and patients to improve care, including The Lancet Haematology Commission on sickle cell disease.[9] This includes twelve key recommendations such as increased genetic screening in babies, access to treatments and education of healthcare professionals. It's my hope that people living with sickle cell disease will start to see a substantial improvement in their experiences of healthcare in the next few years.

Sickle cell disease is one example of patients routinely being unheard by their doctors and healthcare teams, but this happens in many conditions and has been going on for centuries. Doctors are trained to be sceptical of their patients – treating them as unreliable narrators whose testimonies must be doubted. Due to inherent power imbalances, patients have to convince their doctors about the validity of their symptoms to be taken seriously. Minoritised individuals are most likely to be doubted due to stereotypes about their identity, and this exacerbates health inequities, unjust differences in health. Being unheard can lead to significant health consequences such as misdiagnosis, delayed treatment, psychological distress as well as physical harm and death. When patients are repeatedly dismissed and disbelieved, they may silence themselves to avoid further rejection. Such patients are often blamed for not speaking up, but this is difficult and potentially may harm their care further. Instead, healthcare services should take on this responsibility to listen and to make it easier for patients to speak.

*

Doctors have doubted patients' testimonies for a very long time.[10] Professor Daniel Goldberg, a historian of medicine and public health ethicist based at the University of Colorado, wrote about how doctors have historically viewed patients as being possible 'malingerers'. This is defined in the *Cambridge Dictionary* as 'a person who pretends to be ill, in order to avoid having to work'.

Goldberg dates physicians' concerns about malingering to at least a thousand years ago in the West. He describes thirteenth-century physician Arnau de Vilanova as being concerned that patients were trying to trick him by providing urine samples from other people and claiming them as their own. This was being done, he thought, to test his expertise as a physician and potentially discredit him. He listed an incredible *nineteen* pieces of advice for other physicians on how to recognise the genuine patient from the fraudulent. These included recommending physicians 'ask leading questions in the hope the uneducated client would accidentally reveal the real source of the liquid'.

Pain, in particular, has been doubted. Paolo Zacchia, personal physician to several popes and head of the health system in the Papal States, wrote *Quaestiones Medico-Legales*, a medico-legal text published in the seventeenth century. In it, he described groups of people who may falsely claim they are in pain and use this to their advantage. These included 'the armies of the undeserving poor', 'impudent women' and criminal defendants. Goldberg documents how this continued in the West, with certain groups of people more likely to be doubted.

Historically doctors in Europe and America have been white, upper/middle class and male, reflecting innate hierarchical structures in society. This has exacerbated the power imbalance between doctors and patients and engendered a paternalistic approach where the doctor is always right. It also helps explain why people who have traditionally held less power, such as women, the poor and those from racially minoritised groups, are more likely to be deemed untrustworthy. We see this being played out today in many areas of medicine when we look at who is at the sharp end of health inequities.

The power dynamic and inherent doubting of patients has led to doctors thinking theirs is the most important voice in patient interactions, and we see this history playing out today when doctors don't listen to their patients. It is a common problem, despite communication skills being an integral part of a doctor's role. This has been shown in a range of research. The General Medical Council, the professional body that licenses doctors in the UK, found that the persistent failure to listen to patients, failure to explain things to them and to dismiss them are important factors that contribute to poor patient outcomes.[11] A report by the NHS Improvement Patient Safety Initiative Group published in 2018 reviewed evidence about communication in healthcare and found several areas of concern.[12] These included doctors not sharing their decision-making process with patients, dismissing or disbelieving patients, not showing compassion, failing to provide appropriate information or not managing disagreement sensitively. Another study looked at the causes of more than 88,000 patient complaints. The second most common reason for a complaint was poor communication (the first was problems with treatment).[13]

As a doctor, I'll admit I have not always listened to patients as well as I could have. There are incidents that I can remember and almost certainly more I can't. I can give many reasons why I didn't listen – I was hurried, feeling tired, stressed; I missed my lunch due to an overrunning clinic; it was the end of the clinic and my emotional capacity to be fully present had run out; I'd had an argument with a family member or friend; I was having a bad day. I do not mean to use any of these reasons as an excuse for my poor listening, but they do show that I am human and vulnerable to the strains of a demanding job and home life. Am I and the other doctors who don't listen 'bad doctors'? Certainly, some are, but I don't believe this of the majority. In my experience most doctors, including myself, want to do the best we can to help patients get better. This includes hearing them. I agree with doctor and writer Atul Gawande, who said, 'The important question isn't how to keep bad physicians from harming patients; it's how to keep good physicians from harming patients.'[14]

Despite best intentions, miscommunication is pervasive and evidence shows that patients continue to be disappointed. The healthcare system makes it hard for doctors to listen – it is not designed in a way that facilitates careful listening. However, this isn't just an individual or a systemic issue, but ingrained in the way doctors are trained and their approach to medicine. It's even inherent in the language of medicine. Commonly used terms like 'patient denied', 'patient claimed', 'failed treatment', 'poorly com-pliant', 'manipulative' and 'the worried well', can belittle, blame or infantilise patients. This can further disempower patients and damage trust.[15]

While we can be unheard in many areas of our lives, in healthcare it's so important because it can be a matter of life or death.

When we become unwell, being able to communicate and pass on knowledge to others is crucial. We need to tell healthcare profes-sionals about our symptoms, our response to treatment and how we are coping with the illness. When we are unheard this may lead to an incorrect or missed diagnosis, the wrong treatment and dissatisfac-tion with our care. It negatively impacts our relationship with the healthcare team. We may even report feeling gaslighted, being told that our symptoms are 'all in your head'. This can happen to people who are suddenly ill, or to people who have a long-term illness.

A useful concept from philosophy that we can use to understand ways in which people are not heard is that of 'epistemic injustice'. This was coined by Miranda Fricker in 2007 and is defined as a wrong occurring to someone in their capacity as a knower.[16] Being able to produce knowledge and to pass it on to others is a basic human ability, however there are occasions we can't pass knowledge on, because we can't express it in a way the listener can understand, or because they are not receptive to what we are saying. In this we experience an injustice and this is epistemic injustice. Epistemic injustice strikes deep into the heart of how we see ourselves – not being able to convey ourselves to others leaves us feeling less than human. It is at its most damaging when it is cumulative and systematic. Epistemic injustice sits alongside other forms of social injustice that people, particularly those who are minoritised, may experience in different aspects of their lives.

Fricker identified two types of epistemic injustice, although since then, other philosophers have expanded the concept.

The first type is 'testimonial injustice'. This describes how some groups of people, due to stereotypes about their identity, are less likely to be listened to and believed than others. They are viewed as less trustworthy and knowledgeable in what they say and are more likely to be doubted. They experience what Fricker terms a 'credibility deficit'. This most commonly happens to people due to prejudice about their gender, ethnicity, age, class, sexual orientation, ability or religion. For example, this happened to me when I was denied adequate pain relief on the gynaecology ward, probably due to my gender and ethnicity. Very old or younger patients may report being taken less seriously, or people with a working-class accent, or people with a visible disability.

It is easy for testimonial injustice to manifest in healthcare. In medical school, doctors are taught to use mental shortcuts, called heuristics. These help to create and maintain pattern recognition, making diagnosis quicker and easier – a useful and necessary skill. Unfortunately, they are often based on stereotypes. When doctors are rushed or tired (for example the emergency medicine doctor at 4 a.m. who has ten patients waiting to be seen), they may be more likely to rely on heuristics to manage patients. They may become so fixated on a probable diagnosis that they are unable to listen to the individual patient in front of them, and they then carry out the wrong tests. In this way, the patient experiences testimonial injustice. For example, the young gay man who comes to hospital with pain passing urine, due to a kidney stone. The doctor may assume he has a sexually transmitted infection, due to stereotypes reinforced in medical education about gay men having multiple sexual partners. This bias could seriously affect the young man's chances of getting a correct diagnosis. Conversely a 65-year-old woman may come in with pain passing urine due to chlamydia, but may not receive a test due to beliefs that older people are not sexually active.

It's not just people who have a credibility deficit who can be harmed in medicine. Those with a credibility excess, who are seen to be more trustworthy and sincere, have their concerns taken more seriously. They are more likely to be referred for a test. This may lead to over-investigation and unnecessary treatment, which can in turn cause anxiety and be detrimental to their health.

Philosophers Ian James Kidd and Havi Carel also write about how patients are more likely to experience testimonial injustice *because they are ill*. This is particularly the case for those with long-term health conditions. They not only come into contact with healthcare more often but may also experience the stigmatising stereotypes of being a chronically unwell person. These can include being viewed as incapable, confused, incompetent and fundament-ally unable to be objective about their illness. This can make them seem to be unreliable narrators.[17] These negative stereotypes may intersect with others such as racist, ageist or sexist stereotypes and so these patients are particularly vulnerable to testimonial injus-tice. We can see this with our example of sickle cell disease where patients are not heard due to racism and to negative stereotypes about the disease itself.

The other form of epistemic injustice that Fricker describes is that of 'hermeneutical injustice'. This happens when people are unable to communicate their knowledge to healthcare workers in a way that can be understood. This may be directly due to their illness, which impacts their ability to speak or think. Or it may be that the way they explain their symptoms is not in the kind of medical language that the doctor is used to, so they can't understand correctly. Perhaps the patient cannot find the right words, or the right words don't exist, to adequately explain how they are feeling. This is exacerbated when patients are barred from sharing their knowledge as a group, for when patients are not admitted to decision-making boards, their experiences are lost, meaning they cannot take part in healthcare policy-making or allocating resources.[18]

In essence, patients go unheard in healthcare because they are regarded as being untrustworthy and unable to be objective about their illness.

I met Rebecca Tayler Edwards, a development manager at a Disabled People's Organisation when we were both studying for master's degrees in 2022. She contacted me after reading a piece I published on testimonial injustice and went on to write her dissertation focusing on it, entitled 'It's All in Your Head'. She described to me her own experience of seeking healthcare with two invisible, long-term conditions and how it affected her. Rebecca said of doctors, 'You find yourself continually subject to the opinion of one person; who, through their power and position, determines your access to sufficient care, treatment, disability support and credibility in society.' She explained how damaging the cumulative effect of five years of 'dismissal, misdiagnosis, unjust accusal and prejudice' were, wondering if earlier diagnosis and treatment may have improved her physical symptoms. She says the effect on her mental health of being told her symptoms were 'all in her head' is clear – this 'set an unjust precedent to the relationship I have with my body, healthcare professionals and confidence in my own voice'.

I'm very grateful to Rebecca for sharing her personal testimony with me for this book – she highlights the power imbalances between patients and doctors and the effects of being repeatedly unheard. Patients often experience epistemic injustice recurrently and this can silence patients, something I call 'the medical practice of silencing'. What does this look like in real life? Let's consider Hassan's story.

*

Hassan sits quietly on the orange plastic chair in the doctor's office, his foot repetitively tapping the floor, the only outward sign of his anxiety. He's been dreading this appointment with his HIV doctor for the last few weeks. He'd taken the day off from his job in a textile factory and left home early to catch the train to the clinic. As he waved farewell to his wife who was getting the children ready for school, she reminded him that he needed to have an honest conversation with the medical team. But that was easier said than done.

The doctor looks at the computer screen again, frowning. He turns back to Hassan and says, 'Are you sure that everything is OK with your HIV tablets?'

Looking down at his feet, Hassan replies, 'Yes, Dr Greenwood. I take them every day before bedtime just like you tell me to. No problems.'

Noticing his lack of eye contact, the doctor turns his chair to face Hassan and says gently, 'Well, Hassan, the thing is . . . that from the blood tests we took last week, I can see that your HIV viral load, that is the level of virus in the blood, is very high. The number is 801,000 copies. Can you see this here?' He points to the screen.

'Yes, Doctor . . .' Hassan leans in reluctantly, screwing up his eyes to see the small digits on the computer more clearly.

'So, when the HIV medication is working, we expect to see the viral load being very low, less than two hundred copies. But this is very high. And it has been, I can see, for the last year. Do you know why this may be the case?' Dr Greenwood asks.

'Err . . . maybe the tablets stopped working?' Hassan volunteers.

'Well, that's a possibility. Sometimes when people aren't taking their tablets regularly, the HIV virus changes itself and becomes resistant to the medications, so they don't work any more. But when this happens, we don't see such a high viral load level. A level as high as this can only mean that there is no medication in the body . . . is this the case, Hassan? Have you stopped taking your tablets?' Dr Greenwood looks at him inquisitively.

'No, Doctor! I am taking them as you tell me. Every night, two tablets before I go to sleep. None missed,' Hassan protests. He can feel the blood rising to his head and his cheeks start to flush.

Dr Greenwood stares at him for a few seconds that feel like minutes to Hassan. He sighs.

'OK, Hassan. I must tell you that I am worried about these results. When the HIV virus is not under control, it means it can cause damage to your immune system. If this goes on for a while, you may get ill. Do you understand?'

'Yes, Doctor, I understand.' Hassan stares at his feet again.

Dr Greenwood asks, 'Have you had any problems with the tablets? Any side effects?'

Hassan shakes his head. 'No, Doctor. They are good tablets. They go down easily.'

'OK, we need to get to the bottom of this,' Dr Greenwood replies. 'I'm going to get the nurses to do some blood tests and ask the pharmacist to see you. She will ask you some more questions about the tablets and how they are going for you. Take this slip to the receptionist and book to see me in two weeks' time.'

He passes him the blue slip of paper and turns back to his computer to write notes. The consultation is over.

Hassan takes the paper and gets up slowly, making for the door. Holding it ajar, he turns back and says softly, 'Thank you, Doctor. I appreciate it.'

Still facing the computer, Dr Greenwood murmurs, 'OK, I'll see you soon. Take care.' He waits for Hassan to leave the room and types up his consultation notes, documenting the blood results and their discussion. He pauses when he gets to his summary of the problem and shakes his head. He writes, 'Impression: Patient is off his medication, but when asked, denies this. Plan: 1) Blood tests today – drug level to see if any medication in the blood, HIV viral load and resistance test. 2) To see the nurse and pharmacist to discuss his non-compliance further. 3) Review in two weeks with results. If results show no drug in the blood, to have a frank conversation about patient's non-compliance.'

He thinks, feeling exasperated, *Why is Hassan lying to me? I can't help him until he admits he's not taking his meds, and hasn't been for some time. What is the point in not being truthful with me and the rest of the team?'*

He closes the window on the screen with Hassan's notes and starts to prepare for his next patient. It's a busy morning in the HIV outpatient department and he is running late.

Hassan sits in the waiting room, feeling frustrated and sad. He knows that the blood results will show no medication in his blood. He hasn't been taking his tablets for several months. He hadn't wanted to lie to Dr Greenwood, but he felt too ashamed to tell him the truth. When he took the pills, he felt immediately nauseous and once that settled, they disturbed his sleep with the most frightening nightmares. He woke up feeling like he hadn't slept. This constant exhaustion was making it hard to concentrate at work. He had already noticed himself on the verge of dropping off on a shift. At home he was always irritable and snapping at his kids. This was no way to live.

He had tried to talk to Dr Greenwood and the other doctors in the clinic for months about his worries that the tablets were too strong for him. But each time, they told him it would get better, his body would get used to them. He should just put up with the side effects as the tablets were working well.

In the end he stopped trying to tell them, as they just wouldn't listen. One day, as an experiment, he didn't take his tablets. He slept well, waking up feeling refreshed, so he missed them the next night too. A week passed and he felt better than he had in months. He was no longer worried about falling asleep at work. His relationship with his kids had improved. Yes, he was worried about his health in the long-term – HIV was a serious disease, he knew that. But he felt healthy. It was also a relief to take a break from them – they were a daily reminder that he had HIV. When he wasn't taking them, he could almost forget for a short while.

He would try to tell Dr Greenwood the truth the next time, but to be honest, he wasn't sure he would do anything to help. He wondered what it was that made them not take him seriously. Was it his accent or how he spoke? English was his third language and he occasionally struggled to find the words he needed.

*

This is not an uncommon scenario in an HIV clinic and one that I have encountered myself on many occasions as the doctor. Here, the patient has tried to tell his medical team on several occasions that his HIV medications are giving him severe side effects that are causing significant negative impact on his life, at work and at home. He is worried that they are too strong for him and doing him harm. On repeated occasions, when Hassan has tried to talk about this, he has had his concerns dismissed. No one has suggested switching to another drug regimen. No one has reassured him that although he is having serious side effects, the tablets aren't toxic to his body and won't cause him long-term problems. No one has offered him a second opinion. He had to take action himself and stop the tablets. He is aware that in the long term he may be damaging his body, but in the short term, he feels better off the tablets than on them.

So, he stopped telling the doctors what was really going on. He censored himself, telling them what he thought they wanted to hear – that the tablets were fine. Also, he didn't want them to think he was a complainer. Hassan respected his doctors – they knew so much more than he, who had left school at sixteen. And they meant well. He was grateful to the NHS for providing this life-saving treatment free of charge. He wanted to carry on being a 'good patient' in their eyes, so stopped himself from telling his doctors the real issues.

Conversely, the doctor is aware that Hassan is not telling him the truth because his blood tests tell him so. The blood tests don't lie, but as he's been trained to believe, patients do. In his eyes, Hassan is now an unreliable narrator, a patient who cannot be trusted, making him more likely to be disbelieved in the future.

As already mentioned, I have been the frustrated doctor in this scenario on many occasions. It's a situation when as a doctor you may feel *you* are not being heard by the patient who doesn't listen to your advice. It can also shake your confidence in your ability to communicate. Why can't your patient trust you? Over the years I have learnt to understand the viewpoint of patients like Hassan, who have tried to communicate their needs, but with little success. How might the healthcare team have helped Hassan with his predicament?

Firstly, back when he tried to tell his doctors about his side effects, they could have listened better, validated his concerns, reassured him and offered him the option of switching his medication or carrying on. They could have acknowledged that taking medication regularly is not an easy thing for anyone to do, including doctors. I find it hard to finish a course of antibiotics that I have been prescribed for just a week.

It can be particularly difficult for healthcare professionals to understand why some people do not take their HIV treatment regularly as it is life-saving. However, as HIV specialists, we should remember that HIV remains a highly stigmatised condition; taking tablets every day of your life can be difficult, particularly for people who face social and economic adversity, with HIV just one of many daily challenges. The tablets may also act as an unwelcome day-to-day reminder that they have HIV. The medical team could have been more understanding and avoided labelling Hassan a liar, blaming him for not being able to take his medication.

This scenario is an example of what the African American philosopher Kristie Dotson calls 'testimonial smothering'.[19] She describes this as 'the truncating of one's own testimony in order to ensure that the testimony only contains content for which the audience demonstrates testimonial competence'. People who have been disbelieved or dismissed on many occasions want to avoid the trauma of experiencing this again. Instead, they self-censor through silence or by withholding their testimony, as they don't trust the listener to respond appropriately. This silencing of the patient damages the doctor–patient therapeutic relationship and can contribute to mistrust of the healthcare system. Due to previous experiences of rejection, the patient may not trust that their doctor will hear them and take appropriate action.

Globally, research shows adherence to medication is a serious problem. A report by the World Health Organization (WHO) in 2003 found that approximately half of people with long-term illnesses do not take their medicine as prescribed.[20] It stated that improving adherence may have more benefits to people's health than any advances in drug therapy. It's also wasteful – it has been estimated that in the US alone, the cost of drugs not taken may be as much as $100 billion a year.[21] Trust between the patient and the doctor has been reported as being one of the most important parts of supporting patients to adhere to their medication.[22] A study found that where the patient has a very high level of trust in their primary care physician, their rates of adherence are nearly three times higher than those who didn't.[23] It's likely that testimonial smothering, and the repeated experiences of testimonial injustice experienced by patients when they are not heard and believed, may contribute to mistrust and non-adherence to medication. And our response to patients self-censoring their testimony may worsen this mistrust, as we label them as 'unreliable'.

Outside of healthcare, testimonial smothering has been cited by survivors of domestic abuse when describing their interactions with the criminal justice system. Many survivors are deterred from seeking help from the police due to previous experiences of not being believed. In healthcare settings, disclosure of domestic abuse is one area where doctors are intentional about validating the patient's experiences. An integral part of the training for health professionals responding to a disclosure of domestic abuse is to start by saying to the individual, 'I believe you.' If we are more ready to say this in every area of healthcare, along with 'I hear you', we may begin to hear our patients' true testimonies – a crucial step towards being able to identify the care they need.

This sounds simple but is not. Otherwise, perhaps we'd already be seeing an improvement. It will require shifts in the healthcare system, medical training and how doctors view themselves. Language will also need to change so doctors stop using victim-blaming terms like 'non-compliant', and instead start to acknowledge theirs and the healthcare system's role in silencing patients.

*

A common solution offered to patients not being listened to, is that they just need to speak up. I think this is a victim-blaming approach, one that accuses patients of not doing enough to be heard. This can alienate patients further and expands the failure to listen to institutional and structural levels in policy and government.

For example, in 2020 Nadine Dorries, a Minister of State at the Department of Health and Social Care, spoke at the launch of the long-awaited strategy report into endometriosis, the common and under-researched menstrual condition that I've been diagnosed with.[24] When asked about the government's commitment to reducing the eight-year average wait time for an endometriosis diagnosis, Dorries replied, 'Raising the profile is upon all of us.'

She explained: 'That is partly our problem as women – we don't talk enough . . . I think women actually have a responsibility when they go to the GP's practice not to take no for an answer, not to be fobbed off by a doctor. They do not push back, they don't challenge, they're not confident enough to raise an issue, and so they're very easily dismissed.' She went on to say that speaking out is the responsibility of women, as it will make endometriosis a more widely known condition and this will help other women to challenge their doctors.

And it's not just politicians who hold this view. In March 2022, Donna Ockenden, the senior midwife who led on the Ockenden Review into failures of maternity care at Shrewsbury and Telford NHS trust, was being interviewed on the BBC radio show *Woman's Hour*.[25] She said, 'If women have concerns, they must now speak out, they mustn't hold it back, they mustn't sit there thinking well, doctor or midwife knows best, they must question if they are unhappy.'

The presenter Emma Barnett questioned this, saying, 'Patients just want to go to hospital and feel looked after, and now you're saying to question doctors. It's a hard balance to strike.'

This is the power imbalance between doctors and patients that is rooted in Western medicine. It includes the tension between doctors wanting to be respected and patients wanting to be treated with dignity. And often healthcare professionals are not fully aware of their power. In her book *Consumed: A Sister's Story*, writer Arifa Akbar wrote about her sister, Fauzia, who died of undiagnosed tuberculosis.[26] This is an event that shouldn't occur in this day and age as we have the tools to diagnose and treat it. In the book she reflects on the conversations she had with Fauzia's healthcare team and on the power doctors hold: 'Some words were a balm with their accompanying nods and sensitive pauses. Others cut me to the quick... Others continue to sting, however unwittingly the pain may have been inflicted.' When Akbar first met the healthcare team, she was told that 'none of it had been my sister's fault', but at a later meeting that 'her unreliability hadn't helped'. Fauzia had herself spoken about how due to stigma about her mental health conditions, she felt less trusted by the medical team.

There are many reasons why patients and their loved ones or carers do not speak up. It may be due to embarrassment, because they don't want to be seen as 'difficult' or 'complaining'. Certainly, when I was on the ward being denied pain relief, I didn't complain because I was worried that I would be viewed as a nuisance and, due to this, get even worse care. People may not speak up because their expectations of the healthcare team are low, due to previous poor experiences (their own or of people they know), which may have also led to mistrust. Speaking up can even be dangerous for some patients who may get punished for it – for example those who through false stereotypes may be viewed as 'aggressive', like Black men and women. Conversely, patients may trust their healthcare teams too fully, not questioning them, even when they have misgivings about their care.

Patients may also not speak up due to what Hilary Mantel described in her book *Giving Up the Ghost* as 'humble gratitude' to doctors – tidying the house before they arrived to make a good impression.[27] This may seem outdated now, but the power imbalance between patients and doctors is very real and felt by many. My mother, a doctor who worked as a GP in the NHS for forty years and is now retired, tells me that even she 'dresses up' to see her own doctors. She acknowledges that not only does this convey her respect for them, importantly it gives *her* more status. In other words, it boosts her credibility so she will be seen as trustworthy, and therefore heard. For her, this involves needing to overcome a common stereotype of older Asian women – that they are hypochondriacs who complain of physical symptoms that are actually in their head. By dressing up and always managing to get into the conversation that she is doctor, she tries to assert her status as an insider, a member of the medical profession too. Of course, this strategy doesn't always work, as my experience of being a patient in hospital showed.

It's not just my mother who's tried to enhance her credibility in front of doctors. A survey of 3,325 Black Californians found that over a third adjusted their appearance and behaviour to avoid being discriminated against in healthcare. These modifications included 32 per cent reporting they dressed up, 35 per cent changing their speech or how they acted and 41 per cent signalling to doctors that they were educated and knowlededgable.[28]

The risk for patients when they speak up from a place of extreme vulnerability is that they are exposing themselves to a response that may not be positive. I've seen and been part of healthcare teams who become defensive when criticised. Patients or their family are labelled as 'difficult' and this may affect future interactions. I think this particularly happens in healthcare systems that are stretched – healthcare workers feel they are doing their best in an underfunded and understaffed environment, often giving more than they are recognised or paid for. When they are critiqued, I can understand why they may feel sensitive and attacked. Ideally, in healthcare we should, where possible, take feedback as constructive, using it as an opportunity to reflect individually and in teams. When serious incidents occur, these are investigated by hospital teams, who point out failings and make suggestions to avoid these incidents from occurring again. Learning from mistakes, whether they have serious consequences or not, should be embedded in healthcare. Patients and their loved ones have much to teach healthcare professionals. They should be viewed as partners in healthcare.

In 2022, journalist Merope Mills wrote about the avoidable and devastating death of her thirteen-year-old daughter Martha Mills in hospital from sepsis.[29] Martha was admitted with a pancreatic injury having fallen from her bicycle. Merope Mills wrote of her regrets in not asking more questions about her daughter's care. She said that she and her husband had 'blind faith in doctors' and 'had such trust, we feel such fools'. She wrote, 'We tried to be articulate and grateful – these were the experts and we wanted to bring out the best in them. It turns out we were judged in the medical notes: "Mum and Dad pleasant and helpful," reads one entry.' Later in the article she said, 'However indebted you feel to the NHS, don't be afraid to challenge decisions if you have good reason to. It's easy to feel cowed, but hold your ground.' I talked about this article with several of my colleagues who had also read it. While we were all outraged about what had happened to the family, we were familiar with the circumstances that led to Martha's untimely death. Merope Mills is right to say patients and their loved ones should feel like they can speak up and complain.

But some groups of patients are less able to complain than others. Studies looking at who makes patient complaints found that the elderly, patients on lower incomes, less well-educated and those from a racially minoritised group were less likely to complain.[30, 31] It's unlikely that this is because they are getting better care – the more likely explanation is that they feel less able to speak up. This is an issue of health equity – people who are already suffering poorer health outcomes are less able to complain about worse healthcare and are blamed for it.

*

'Doctor, doctor! People keep ignoring me.'
   'Next please.'

'Doctor,' says the patient, 'whenever I get up from my sleep, for half an hour I feel dizzy, and then I'm all right.' And the doctor says, 'Get up half an hour later, then.'

Doctor! Doctor! jokes highlighting the humorous side of doctor–patient miscommunication have been around since Roman times. The joke I've cited above about dizziness appeared in *The Philogelos* (or *Laughter Lover*), a Roman joke book which experts believe was probably written in the fourth or fifth centuries AD.[32]

However, as we know well, doctor–patient communication is rarely a laughing matter, and this shows that the problem has existed for millennia. The effects of poor communication can be profound, damaging the doctor–patient relationship and causing preventable harm to patients. My experience as a patient profoundly changed the way I practice medicine and communicate with patients. This is something many doctors who have experienced being on the other side of healthcare go through. We find that it's a shock not to be listened to, our credibility questioned even as an insider. It shouldn't be this way, of course – doctors should be able to show compassion without the lived experience of being a patient.

It is estimated that every thirty-six hours, there are a million contacts between patients and healthcare staff in the NHS.[33] This represents a million opportunities for communications to go wrong, but also a million opportunities for positive interactions, which can make patients feel safer and more secure. Being heard and validated gives us dignity. When we are ill, we are already in a situation where we feel undignified. This may be through wearing the uniform of the sick, the hospital gown, or when we suffer the indignity of no longer being in control of our body due to illness. If we are not heard in healthcare, we lose some of our humanity.

This is the opposite of what the vast majority of people working in healthcare are aiming for. Most healthcare professionals go into their jobs with good intentions to help people, not to make them feel worse. And yet, this still happens, despite those good intentions. You may be wondering, *What can patients do to be better heard?* This is an important question and I make some suggestions overleaf. I intend these actions to be empowering and to help patients take control in an imperfect healthcare system. However, I provide them with an important caveat – I strongly believe that the onus should be on healthcare to change, not on patients who are dealing with enough difficulty already.

How individual patients (perhaps you?) can be better heard in healthcare

Plan for your consultation

This can include writing down how you have been feeling, any new symptoms or updates on your condition, your current medications. Bring any information you may have received about other medical appointments or investigations, such as scan results. Think about what questions you have and write them down. You can refer to these during the consultation so you can ensure you have asked them by the end.

This can be difficult if you are attending hospital for an emergency, but bringing even your regular medications with you can help. This saves the medical team from calling your GP to find this out, something that may not be possible when the surgery is closed. I've admitted patients from the emergency department on a Friday night and not been able to get a list of medication until Monday morning when their GP surgery opened. This has been frustrating for the patient and the medical team.

Importantly, it also shows the medical team that you are knowledgeable and take your health seriously – something that may help them take *your* care more seriously.

Write things down

During the appointment, write down what you hear. This will not only help you to remember afterwards what has been discussed from your point of view, but helps during the appointment. If you are writing things down that you don't understand, ask the doctor to explain further.

I often find myself in the position of noting down diagnoses and medications for my patients to take away – I always appreciate the opportunity to do so, and often offer to whether the patient accepts this or not.

Ask for sources of information

Ask the doctor if they have any leaflets or recommended websites for you to look at when you leave the consultation room. It's easy to do an internet search of medical conditions and be faced with alarming amounts of disinformation or information that is not relevant to you. Healthcare professionals will often have a list of resources that they believe are reliable and easy to understand – ask them for their recommendations.

Reputable sites from the UK include:

- www.patient.info
- www.nhs.uk
- www.healthtalk.org

Bring a friend with you

Having a friend or relative present means that they can advocate for you. Tell them before the consultation what you want to get out of it. They can ask questions when you are not able to and may remember parts of the conversation that you have forgotten. Consultations are emotional and often news is delivered that can be surprising, complex or difficult to process – this makes it harder to remember exactly what's been said.

Bringing a friend means that you have an observer and someone who can stick up for you. While this may have got harder to do with the advent of COVID-19 and the increase in telephone or video consultations, in most situations patients can ask to be seen face to face and to bring an advocate. However, a friend or relative should not be used as a translator – you can request a trained translator. You should also be happy for them to hear about your personal details – consider whether there is something you don't want them to know about you. If so, let them know that you may ask them to step out of the consultation at times.

Consider asking to see the same doctor

Having a doctor who you have seen before can be helpful for you both. It means that you already have a relationship so you may be more comfortable conversing. They will also be familiar with your medical history so you don't need to start from the beginning.

(Of course, this is only useful if you had a good experience – if not, ask to see someone else!)

Name the problem

'I don't feel you are hearing what I'm saying.'

'I don't think you are taking my problems seriously.'

It can be scary to do this as you may be worried that this will annoy the doctor and be detrimental for your care. Sadly, I cannot guarantee this won't happen. However, in general doctors want to feel they have helped their patients. By telling them that there is a communication problem, it will hopefully encourage them to take a different and more successful approach. If, however, this causes antagonism, then knowing how to raise your concern to a higher level is essential. Having a friend with you may help you feel braver to speak up, or they may speak up for you if you're unable.

Know your rights

As a patient you are legally entitled to good-quality care. This can include asking for a second or even third opinion – doctors should not be offended by this, as they do this informally and formally all the time, particularly with complex cases.

You are also entitled to ask for a copy of your results or medical notes if you want them.

All healthcare settings will have a process of how to complain or give feedback that should be clearly visible to patients – make sure you know where to find this. For example, hospitals in England have a Patient Advice and Liaison Service (PALS), which provides a point of contact for patients, their carers and families. Many patient organisations can also advise on this.

Educate yourself on your condition

This is not essential as sometimes it may feel overwhelming, but it can help. You will become more familiar with the medical terms around your diagnosis and treatment. It may also help you use language that doctors are familiar with, making it easier for them to hear and understand you.

Ask who is in charge

You will have someone who has overall responsibility for your care (often a senior doctor such as a consultant or GP). If you feel you are not having your concerns addressed adequately, ask to speak to them. It's their duty to listen to you and ensure you are as satisfied as you can be with your treatment.

Let them know if you have special communication needs

If English is not your main language, or you have other issues with communication, let your doctors know in advance. They can arrange for your needs to be accommodated, such as ensuring an interpreter is present.

Summary: How individual patients (perhaps you?) can be better heard in healthcare

- Plan for your consultation.
- Write things down in the consultation.
- Ask for reputable sources of information.
- Bring a friend with you.
- Consider asking to see the same doctor.
- Name the problem if you are not being heard.
- Know your rights.
- Educate yourself on your condition.
- Ask who is in charge of your care.
- Let them know if you have special communication needs.

2

Devalued

Why Doctors Don't Listen

I can remember getting my first complaint from a patient as if it were yesterday.

I was walking to work through the local market, my mind on the day ahead. It was going to be a busy one – clinic, ward round, meetings. I was counting the weeks until the end of the year and some time off. As I stood at the pedestrian crossing waiting for the light to turn green, I idly flicked through my phone, refreshing my social media apps and my work email account. At the top was an email from our clinic manager, forwarding me the complaint.

As I read it, my first reaction was that the patient had got me confused with another doctor. I didn't recognise the person it described, let alone believe it could be me. The complaint described a doctor who was condescending, who didn't take a patient's wishes into account, or work with them to find the best and most suitable management plan for them. A doctor who didn't listen. It just didn't feel like me. Denial and shame hit me like twin missiles to the chest, momentarily taking my breath away. The remaining journey to work was a daze.

As soon as I got to my office, I frantically looked up the electronic notes from our last consultation, finding nothing I had documented which suggested an awkward or difficult encounter. And it didn't stick out in my memory, like some consultations do. Clearly, I had not been sensitive enough to the patient's emotions and did not pick up on their discomfort. Looking back further into the records, I found that the patient had made complaints about several colleagues over the years. I felt relieved. This was obviously a 'difficult' patient who had excessive expectations which no doctor could hope to meet. This notion was reinforced when I debriefed to my colleagues. They too expressed surprise in the complaint and its nature. This was also a relief: my colleagues, some of whom I'd worked with for most of my career, knew that this was not the doctor *I really was.*

But I had a niggling thought – my personal experience wasn't that the patient was 'difficult'. I had been their doctor for several years, and we had, I thought, a reasonable relationship. They were always personable with me, and we had even shared moments of humour. I knew they found coming into clinic to be highly nerve-wracking so I consciously prepared for this, doing everything I could to make it a bit less stressful. To my knowledge we'd not had any significant disagreements before.

So, although this was a patient that could be (and had been) easily labelled 'difficult', this wasn't my experience of them. I had to take responsibility for my role in what upset them. And that was what made accepting the complaint harder – I liked to think of myself as a doctor who acknowledges the momentous nature of a clinic appointment for a patient, who tries to adjust my language and my posture to reduce power imbalances, who tries to listen to and work with patients. To essentially make the patient leave the clinic feeling like they matter and that their needs are important enough to have been heard and taken seriously. This was reflected in some of my patient feedback over the years. But that's not what this patient experienced. So, *who* was the doctor that the patient saw that day? How could I bridge the gap between the doctor I and my colleagues thought I was, and the one the patient described? Maybe I had been clumsy with my communication, and what I said was open to a wide range of interpretation? Maybe I'd been having a bad day? Or worse, was I the doctor I feared becoming, worn down and cynical by years of working in an under-resourced healthcare system? Can these images even be reconciled? Perhaps the patient had misunderstood what I said, or was even wanting to be hurtful, as some co-workers suggested.

An older colleague wisely told me to view the complaint as something to be expected in our roles. Most doctors will get a complaint at least once in their careers. A 2021 survey of British doctors by the Medical Defence Union found that 97 per cent of GPs and 88 per cent of hospital consultants have had at least one complaint from a patient.[1] Although upsetting and occasionally unfair, they are always an opportunity to reflect on our practice and to learn. Whatever had happened, the patient did not leave the consultation feeling cared for, and that mattered.

Several months after the complaint, I had enough distance to reflect on my reaction to it. My first instinct had been to become defensive, trying to prove to myself and to others that I wasn't a bad doctor. I then came to understand that despite my good intentions, I wasn't the doctor that the patient needed on that day. It was never my plan to be a poor listener. When I started medical school, I had every intention of listening to my patients' concerns with empathy, eliciting the salient details to make a diagnosis and treat them. How did I go from this laudable aim to being a doctor who didn't listen?

I want to understand why doctors (like me) don't listen, why we dismiss patients, and how we can silence them. Of course, it is inevitable that mistakes can happen in our interactions, however it's how we reflect and respond to our failures that is most important. We also have to consider that some of this is structural – we don't work in environments that prioritise listening, so time and space is limited. Like the rest of society, we may hold bias against certain groups of people which means we may take what they say less seriously. However, during my research I came across an unexpected finding. I grew to realise that much of our practices of not hearing and of silencing patients are actually ingrained in our profession – true listening can be challenging and even make us question our role as doctors. This was difficult for me to face, and I wonder how it will feel for doctors and other healthcare professionals reading this book. It is important that we do not look away; we need to accept this, however uncomfortable it is, and work to address it. For patients reading this, I hope you see that doctors, in the majority, want to do the best for their patients, however sometimes we are fighting a flawed system to do so. We start to see this in medical school, where we learn the medical practice of silencing at the very start of our careers.

*

I have happy memories of the summer before I started medical school in 1998. It was a haze of lie-ins, hanging out with friends, going to festivals and talking about our future. We were on the precipice of the rest of our lives. I can still feel that excitement now, the prospect of leaving home in suburban Essex for central London, to live independently and make new friends. Even going shopping with my parents to buy kitchen essentials and stationery was a thrill. Most importantly I was going to learn a profession – in just six years, I'd be graduating as a fully trained doctor. I'd be like the doctors I'd seen on the telly in countless shows – *Casualty, Cardiac Arrest* – impressive, confident and knowledgeable.

Medical school did not disappoint. The first year of lectures were like learning a new language; we were taught the basics of anatomy, pathology, physiology, pharmacology – essentially how the body worked and what happened when things went wrong. With my fellow students, we encountered tutors who did their best to enthuse us on duller topics; a favourite was a professor who made sound effects to illustrate the intimate workings of the human cell (his performance of a cell dividing remains... memorable). There were also those that made no effort to interact with us during long, monotonous lectures where we passed notes to entertain ourselves. I still have some of these and they remain a hilarious reminder of those years before we had mobile phones with which to message each other.

Together, we faced our fear of being singled out in seminars by tutors who believed in humiliation as a teaching method. And I can remember our collective apprehension of practical anatomy classes as we started the year. We'd meet nervously in the anatomy lab every week wearing white coats and speaking in hushed voices, trying not to breathe in the smell of embalming chemicals that pervaded the space too deeply. We were divided up into small groups and assigned a cadaver to dissect. We were told that these were people who had donated their bodies after death to science, so that we could learn from them. The reverence with which we approached these sessions helped me understand that we were embarking on a career of great privilege. We would be entrusted with people's most private secrets, and this was something to be respected.

These initial experiences bound us closely together as a group. We were starting to enjoy our status as 'medical students' – separate to, and we believed slightly superior to, other university students. After all, we'd achieved the highest grades to get on the course and we were learning a subject that *mattered* – we were going to save lives and that made us important in our eyes. Our hours were longer than everyone else's so we didn't have much opportunity to socialise with students on other courses. My best friends at university, who I remain friends with to this day, were those from my course who I shared accommodation with in the first year. We'd been placed in university halls on the opposite side of London to our campus, and so left early each day to cross the city, a complicated route that involved a bus and two tube trains. I can remember tiptoeing through the corridors so as not to wake my neighbours who didn't have such an early start. I'd meet my friends at the bus stop and we'd catch up on the gossip from the night before or compare assignment answers.

I share these memories to explain how medical school instilled in us a sense of being different from other students – it made us think we were special, a feeling that was reflected by our environment, and that we reinforced in ourselves and each other. This contributed to a sense of hubris, something that follows many doctors into their working lives. Hubris is an excessive pride that can discourage the humility that is required to listen well. It encourages a paternalistic attitude to patients, which shifts the power balance in our direction. *We, as doctors, know more than you and so know what's best for you.* It may also give us an air of superiority, which makes us seem unapproachable and unsympathetic. I was once gifted a mug bearing the words, 'Please do not confuse your Google search with my medical degree'. While this is meant to be humorous, it makes an important point – we doctors think we know best, and it is only our knowledge that counts. What is missed is the most fundamental understanding that without patients – or those kind people who donated their bodies to science – there would be no doctors.

The lack of contact with students from other healthcare professions such as nursing, physiotherapy, occupational therapy and dietetics also contributed to our hubris. Knowing that we would eventually be the people making the most difficult life-or-death decisions meant that we knew our place was destined to be at the top of the medical hierarchy. This order is ingrained in the healthcare workforce and can have negative impacts on patient safety. People lower in the hierarchy may feel less able to speak up and question a management plan – they dare not query senior doctors even if they suspect there is something wrong. This clearly needs to change, and perhaps by meeting our healthcare colleagues at university, we will become more used to seeing them as our equals, with similar but separate roles and skills that they bring to patient care.

The empathy with which we started medical school also began to be replaced with what medical student and writer Xi Chen calls 'medicine's hidden curriculum of brutal pragmatism'. He describes this as a 'reliance on derogatory humor towards patients, the ever-present (and increasing) exhaustion of its staff, and the overwhelming sensation of being surrounded by suffering but only being liable for the selfish act of learning'.[2] Research shows that as they go through medical school, students lose their empathy. The reasons for this have been described as increasingly stressful workloads and the prioritisation of biomedical knowledge over a more holistic approach to care (treating the disease rather than the patient).[3] In other words, as students, we learn to harden ourselves, creating boundaries which mean that as we enter our working lives, we can remain detached from our patients and continue to function. While these boundaries are important, they shouldn't mean the absence of warmth, listening or understanding. This is also where we learnt to doubt what patients tell us – we were taught that we could not always trust their testimonies.

As the years progressed, we went from memorising facts to

learning how to apply them in practice. This was the beginning of our understanding of the art of medicine. We started to have 'Communication Skills' sessions integrated in our timetables, where we practised how to take a patient history and to explain a diagnosis and treatment. Taking a history was taught in a formulaic fashion, using a framework. There were set questions, to ask in a set order. The core of these included the patient's 'presenting complaint' (why they had come to the doctor), the history of the presenting complaint (the background as to why they had come), past medical history (previous and current health conditions), drug history (medications and allergies), family history (any conditions that ran in the family) and finally their 'social history'. This encompassed everything else about a patient's life that may be pertinent to making a diagnosis, such as whether they smoked, drank alcohol, took drugs, what job they did, who they lived with, whether they had recently travelled abroad, and so on.

We were taught to start with open questions: 'What's brought you here today?' and to move on to closed questions: 'Are you bringing up blood when you cough?' By doing this, we could sift through the information given to us, working out what was useful and what was irrelevant. This meant we could reject some diagnoses, consider others and know what to ask next. We narrowed diagnostic options further and further until just a few remained. By doing this we learnt to recognise diagnostic patterns. This was important as we could collect information at speed and control what the patient told us – a skill we required to make sure we would be efficient. However useful this skill is, one critique of this data-processing approach is that it may overlook some of the patient's humanity, and by doing so, take away our own. We missed the opportunity to just listen, to find out a patient's life story, *who* they were outside of the hospital, as a fellow human and not just as a patient. This is information that may give us a better idea of their concerns, their motivations and their priorities. These are all useful for their future management, not just their diagnosis.

A study published in 1984, observing doctor–patient consultations in the United States, showed that on average it took just eighteen seconds for a doctor to interrupt a patient's presenting complaint.[4] The patient was only able to finish stating their concerns in less than a quarter of the consultations. The authors concluded that this selective mode of history taking, with the early use of closed questions, can potentially miss much useful information from the patient. I take these findings with several caveats – this is a one-off study that was done almost forty years ago in the United States, so the results may be out of date, or not transferrable to most doctor–patient consultations. However, it does highlight that focused history taking, which may be regarded as more efficient, might actually not be. It may not help us get all the data we need to make an effective management plan. And letting patients finish what they have to say may not take as much time as we fear. Another study where doctors let patients tell their whole presenting complaint without interruption, showed they usually stopped after an average time of only ninety-two seconds.[5] This should leave enough time for doctors to dig into the important parts in more detail, even in a ten-minute consultation.

Medical students are often regarded by patients as being very good listeners. Ironically it is their inexperience that is so valued by patients. They have not yet learnt how to be selective with their questioning so everything the patient says is potentially important. This is something they unlearn as they become more experienced and efficient with history taking. We also learn as students that taking a history is an honour. When sharing their history, patients are asking for help, displaying their vulnerability. To be trusted with these most private thoughts and concerns is a great privilege. Sometimes this can get overlooked in the stressful working conditions of a hospital or surgery, where it can feel like the most important thing is getting through the shift and seeing as many patients as safely as possible. But I think that this appreciation is not lost; sometimes we just need the opportunity to reflect on it and celebrate it.

The last three years of medical school involved clinical placements, where we were attached to medical teams on wards for our experiential learning – attending ward rounds, practising history-taking and examination skills with real patients, and then learning how to present our findings concisely to our colleagues. We rotated through surgery, general medicine, paediatrics, obstetrics and gynaecology, general practice; sometimes being placed in hospitals outside of London for weeks at a time. This was exciting as it was closer to what we would be doing on a daily basis in our future jobs, but also terrifying. It was more embarrassing to be observed by your peers to be asking a patient about a symptom in a clumsy way, than to not know an anatomical term when asked.

End of year exams, which were previously just written papers testing our memory for facts, began to include a practical assessment of our clinical and communication skills. This was called the Objective Structured Clinical Examination (OSCE) and this continues to be a method used to examine doctors in training and in post-graduate exams. My last OSCE was in 2012 for the Diploma in HIV Medicine, eight years after I qualified. My non-medical friends couldn't believe I was still revising for these so far into my career. At my university, OSCEs consisted of up to twelve 'stations' where we'd encounter a different scenario – for example, examining the abdomen of a mannequin, taking a medical history from a patient-actor who reports a headache, measuring blood pressure, pretending to take blood from a plastic arm. In the corner of the station sat the examiner, holding a clipboard on which there was a marking scheme. In OSCEs, some patients are played by trained actors, who also contribute to the scoring, grading the student on whether they are personable and professional.

We dreaded OSCEs the most. However much we prepared, we could be undone by our nerves. The term 'role-play' still strikes fear into my heart. Now I regularly find myself examining students and post-graduate doctors and I see how scary candidates find these scenarios. Even I feel nervous, as an examiner I am keen to make sure I give the examinees as fair a go as possible. OSCEs are a rite of passage for doctors, one we all have to learn to get through. The stations that made us the most apprehensive were those where we weren't just collecting information from a patient, for example ones where we need to discuss the pros and cons of a treatment. There was always a station in which we anticipated an uncomfortable conversation. These included 'breaking bad news' such as telling a patient they had a cancer diagnosis, or that of the 'difficult or angry patient/relative' where our task was to calm them down and defuse the situation.

I now realise that these were some of the most important skills to learn. Our tutors did not tell us that in real life many of our interactions would be uncomfortable or complex, not a minority. Medical school taught us that we should expect to spend much of our working lives treating what I call 'the ideal patient'. These expectations are guided by socially accepted norms of how people should look and act when unwell. However, the 'ideal patient' doesn't exist. For many reasons, few people fit into the box of how we are taught a patient may behave when unwell. They may not speak English as their first language; they may not explain their symptoms in medical terms we are used to; their anxiety about what's wrong with them may affect the way they answer our questions; they may not understand what we are asking; they may not follow our medical advice; they may feel a pressure to look like they are in control; they may be scared about showing their vulnerability; they may be feeling emotionally detached or numbed; they may be worried that they are coming across as too dramatic. Their reactions may be different from expected due to the culture they are from, or if they are neurodiverse. They may also be worried about potential discrimination, which may make them feel the need to act more composed than they feel. Patients are people, individuals with real lives outside of their illness, with stories gathered over a lifetime – they do not fit into neat boxes of how we expect them to be. When patients do not appear as expected, they will start to be doubted and a doctor may even suspect that they are being deceived or manipulated.

I can remember once seeing a patient in the emergency department where I worked, who came in with the symptoms of a heart attack. The way he described them was exactly like I had read in my medical textbooks. Recognising this, we quickly performed an electrocardiogram, which confirmed the diagnosis and we were able to treat him immediately with clot-busting drugs. As he was recovering, I asked him whether he had a medical background, as he appeared extremely familiar with medical terminology. He replied that he didn't, but as an actor he had played patients in OSCEs countless times over the years and picked up some terms. In this real-life scenario, he was the 'ideal patient', which meant we recognised his pattern of symptoms quickly and were able to treat him straight away. Such a case is the exception.

When patients do not respond in the way we have been taught to expect, as an 'ideal patient', we may label them 'poor historians'. But perhaps it's us as doctors who are 'poor history takers'? If we were taught to acknowledge that the ideal patient does not exist, this would have prepared us better for being doctors. British psychiatrist Dr Chloe Beale has written that 'Realism and honesty should be embedded in training, rather than teaching perfect medicine in an imperfect world.'[6] I would go further and say that realism, honesty *and* empathy should be embedded in our training. We should teach how social and economic inequality can impact patients' health and their interactions with doctors, how we can have healthy boundaries while connecting with each patient we see and how we should be committing our time to listening and openness just as we do to data and diagnosis. By teaching this we could develop doctors who are less paternalistic and dismissive, more open to hearing what patients tell them, and who are more likely to support rather than blame them for their decisions.

We must also consider how bias affects our interactions with patients. Our society is riddled with bias, and our healthcare system is certainly not immune from it. Certain prejudice is inherent in society and doctors are part of this society, so may hold the same prejudices. As previously discussed, due to testimonial injustice, patients from minoritised groups are more likely to experience a credibility deficit due to their gender, age, ability, ethnicity, class, sexual orientation or religion. This leads to them being dismissed and disbelieved. Bias can be explicit and there are some doctors who are aware that they discriminate against certain social groups – they should be disciplined for this. Unconscious bias is more common and harder to address, because people may not be aware they hold prejudicial views, and that they treat some people differently to others.

An important tool to guide our judgements on credibility is humility. By being open to information that we don't know, we validate the speaker as our equal. This encourages them to speak, as we come across as being non-judgemental. We may also learn from them, which may in turn widen our knowledge and perhaps even change some of our attitudes. Psychotherapist Carl R. Rogers wrote in 1952 that 'Listening with understanding means taking a very real risk . . . you run the risk of being changed yourself'.[7] Patients know their bodies and conditions better than anyone else, and should be regarded as having this expertise. By being humble, curious and listening with understanding, I think we can start to overcome some of our internal biases and make more accurate judgements about a patient's credibility. We may perpetrate less testimonial injustice by doing so.

Doing this well will not be easy. In her book, *The End of Bias: How We Change Our Minds,* Jessica Nordell writes about how when we are made aware of our own biases, we can become defensive and feel shame.[8] These are barriers that must be overcome in order for us to change. To do this we must be willing to challenge ourselves with compassion and commit to the uncomfortable process that is required to truly change. We also need to recognise the circumstances when we are more likely to rely on stereotypes. This can happen more commonly when we are tired or stressed. Acknowledging this may help us to reflect on our decisions at these times. Are we making judgements based on the individual in front of us, or on a stereotypical assumption of them we have in our minds?

While individual reflection and change is important, institutional solutions that take away opportunities for bias may be more effective. Healthcare services can use tools such as policies and proformas to overcome individual bias. An example of this comes from my specialty: in 2022, hospitals in London received funding to introduce opt-out HIV (and hepatitis B and C) testing to adults attending their emergency departments. One rationale for this was that people diagnosed with HIV were often not tested until the disease had progressed, worsening their prognosis. Look-back reviews showed that these people had often been seen in healthcare settings in the year before diagnosis and not been offered a test. The doctors they had seen did not feel they fit the picture of who they believed would get HIV. Anyone can get HIV, but persisting stereotypes suggest it is only certain types of people who are affected and this contributes to stigma. By offering the test to everyone, it takes out the need for individual healthcare workers to make value judgements about whether a person fits the stereotype. This scheme has proved to be successful with more than 80 people newly diagnosed in the first 100 days.[9] Another example is the Alliance for Innovation on Maternal Health's patient safety bundles.[10] These are evidence-based guidelines that standardise the clinical response to common causes of preventable maternal mortality, such as very high blood pressure. The bundles place equity at their core and again show how a systematic solution can defeat doctor bias and lead to effective change.

While we wait for a fundamental cultural shift in societal attitudes towards minoritised populations, to overcome prejudice and bias in the healthcare service both individual and institutional strategies are needed. These will help to ensure that the people who need to be heard most by their doctors, will be.

*

Why do doctors think they don't listen? I asked colleagues from different areas of medicine this question and this is a selection of the answers I received.

- 'My clinic was running late and I was worried that I still had ten people to see after this patient.'
- 'I needed to be quick. I couldn't find a private room in the department, and had to talk to the patient in the corridor.'
- 'My mind was thinking ahead to what I needed to ask the patient, and listing what tests I needed to order, so I wasn't very present.'
- 'I was distracted by the patient's child who was jumping on and off the weighing scales, and I was worried they would break them.'

- 'I'd had an argument with my partner before coming to work, and my mind kept going back to it.'
- 'There was no interpreter booked, so it was difficult to communicate.'
- 'Our appointments are ten minutes long. The patient had come with multiple issues and I only had time to discuss one or two.'
- 'The patient was talking about their chronic back pain again. I had already investigated it and made the appropriate referrals. I wasn't sure what else I could add.'
- 'I still had the patient from the previous consultation in my mind, thinking about whether I had made the right management plan.'
- 'It was coming to the end of clinic and I had already seen fifteen patients that morning. I was hungry and hadn't slept well the night before.'
- 'The patient had come in asking for a specific treatment that I had already said probably wouldn't work. There was no point going over this again.'
- 'The patient had internet searched their symptoms and found a lot of irrelevant and scary explanations for what could be causing their problem. I was trying to reassure them in the time we had, but I couldn't stop them talking.'
- 'The patient had a known chronic condition and was already under the specialist team. There wasn't anything more I could do to help.'
- 'The receptionist called me in the middle of the consultation to let me know about another issue.'
- 'We'd had some difficult consultations in the past and I was nervous about today's, which meant I may not have been as present as I could have been.'
- 'It was unclear from what the patient was telling me, what the problem actually was.'
- 'I had an email pop up on my screen, which distracted me.'

This small sample demonstrates a variety of reasons for why doctors may not listen to their patients. Some of them are outside of their control. Many show that doctors are human, and will have some days when they are better at listening than others. After all a typical clinic session can include seeing a huge variety of patients and conditions, with a wide scope of knowledge needed to come up with management plans at speed. Doctors have to see a patient and then reset, wiping their minds clean so they are refreshed and open to hearing the next patient. They must do this numerous times a day. I have met plenty of doctors who are excellent at listening to their patients, and enjoy this as an essential part of their jobs. However, maintaining this in every consultation is hard, despite good intentions to do so.

Whatever the cause for not listening well, doctors should always be aware that for a patient the consultation may be hugely important. They may be in a high state of anticipation having waited weeks or even months to see us. They may be worried that their symptoms will reveal they have a life-changing illness and if so, how they will cope? For doctors, the patient will be one of many they see that day. In general practice in the UK it's not uncommon for doctors to see over forty patients a day. Consultations are a routine part of daily work life. Doctors must acknowledge this difference in expectations so we can, where possible, try to meet them.

To do this, we need to create the conditions in which doctors are better able to listen. This includes time, space and prioritising listening. It is hard to listen when you are in a busy department struggling to hear the patient's voice above the hubbub outside your cubicle. For patients, it is difficult to talk about the most private of matters at the bedside with just curtains around it for privacy. On countless occasions I've had to hold serious conversations with patients and their families in the ward staff room, as it was the only private space we could find. Building physical environments that encourage deeper conversations would really help doctors listen. This could include rooms dedicated to private conversations, and having some with softer furnishings that look less clinical, making a patient feel more comfortable to talk.

Doctors also need time to listen. As healthcare systems around the world become busier, productivity has been emphasised. This discourages listening even when we want to, creating a tension between using our interpersonal skills which make the day more enjoyable, and completing our tasks in a short time frame. Ten minutes per consultation (which is the time given for most GPs in the UK) is just not long enough. We also need breaks built in to our working days. This often doesn't happen as we take advantage of any 'free time' to get on with endless administrative tasks. I am guilty of this too – eating a sandwich at my desk and choosing to answer emails or check blood results when I should be stepping away. I have a colleague who advocates going out for a short walk at lunchtime, but despite my best intentions I never do it.

Researchers have looked into the impact that not having breaks has on decision-making by judges. They found that judges were more likely to make favourable decisions in court after they had taken a short break for food. Before their breaks they were more likely to make 'safe' decisions that went with the status quo.[11] They termed this the 'hungry judge' effect, a form of decision fatigue which I think is relevant to doctors. We are more likely to make conservative treatment plans and offer unnecessary prescriptions as the path of least resistance when we are in need of a break.[12] Perhaps by ensuring short breaks are incorporated in long clinic lists, giving doctors time to breathe, they may feel more able to make decisions that aren't swayed by tiredness and hunger.

In the NHS, financial incentives are often given to organisations to encourage them to be more productive. But listening is not valued by policymakers in this way. Productivity is often measured as the number of tests, diagnoses and treatments made, rather than the quality of consultations. While this may seem efficient, it doesn't recognise consultations where the act of listening is in itself therapeutic and tests and treatments are not required. Instead, they could use other measurements such as the Consultation and Relational Empathy (CARE) Measure, a patient questionnaire developed by researchers at the Universities of Glasgow and Edinburgh.[13] This includes questions like 'How good was the doctor at really listening?' and 'How good was the doctor at letting you tell your story?'[14] There are also methods developed for hospital services to encourage patients to feedback on their experience of care. These include Patient-Reported Experience Measures (PREMs), which ask patients about the quality of the information they were provided with, the level of their trust in staff, as well as waiting times and clinic environment.[15]

The healthcare systems we work in are designed in a way that actively discourages listening. Doctors and patients lose some of their humanity in these conditions, leaving both feeling unheard. It's not just *where* or *how* we work though, it's a more fundamental issue about what we believe our role as doctors to be, and there is much debate as to what role we should take. What is beneficial for patients and doctors may be at odds with what is seen to be beneficial for healthcare systems.

*

The role of the GP in the UK was cemented early on in *A Fortunate Man: The Story of a Country Doctor*, widely regarded as a classic of medical literature and often recommended to medical students.[16] Published in 1967, it is a moving portrait of a family doctor, John Sassall. He invited writer John Berger and photographer Jean Mohr to stay with him and his family for six weeks and shadow him while he attended to his patients. Through intimate photos and writing, they document Sassall's work life, providing the reader with philosophical reflections on the role of the doctor as healer. It is often regarded as a love letter to a type of medical practice that is much rarer now. Sassall was a well-known member of his small rural community, and was always available for his patients. His work was all-consuming. Berger wrote, 'Like an artist, or like anybody else who believes that his work justifies his life, Sassall – by our society's miserable standards – is a fortunate man.' He was able to witness the many possibilities of human experience, but watching from such close range, at times, 'the suffering of his own patients and his own sense of inadequacy' was overwhelming. Although it was published more than fifty years ago, it serves as a reminder that medicine is more than just doling out drugs – it is about treating the whole person.

Traditionally, a family doctor would know a person over their lifetime and look after their relatives. As an integral part of the local community, they would also have a good understanding of the issues important to it. In the UK, the Royal College of General Practitioners was created in 1952 to improve standards and raise the profile of family doctors. They emphasised that GPs were experts in their field, one that has its own specific art and knowledge. This was a speciality that valued talking and listening to patients as much as clinical examination, and this was just as important as the other more drama-filled, heroic aspects of medical practice.[17] General practice continues to be one of the few medical specialities that encourages training in communication skills after medical school, with trainee GPs having their consultations videotaped for reflection afterwards.

In 2022, journalist Polly Morland and photographer Richard Baker's *A Fortunate Woman: A Country Doctor's Story* was published, and it can be seen as a companion piece to *A Fortunate Man*.[18] They focus on GP Rowena Christmas, who is now working in John Sassall's former surgery. As well as being a beautiful depiction of the life of a contemporary country doctor, it is a fascinating comparison of medical practice in the 1960s to modern day. Now, as then, the importance of continuity of care shines through. Morland writes, 'Put simply, she is a doctor who knows her patients. She is the keeper of their stories, over years and across generations, witness to the infinite variety of their lives.' Morland describes Dr Christmas' focus on her patients, giving them the time they need to talk about what is wrong. One of the patients in the waiting room remarked, 'the point is she's a person, not a service. That's why she's always late for appointments. It's because she spent time with the one before you. And, if you ask me, that's a very good thing.'

However, an underlying theme of *A Fortunate Woman* is that this is a form of medical practice that may soon no longer exist. The doctor–patient relationship is under threat from inadequate resourcing, changes to clinical practice and the nature of the workforce. The population is growing and getting older due to medical and social advances. This means there are more people with complex health needs who require a regular review with their GP. However, there are now fewer doctors, which makes this difficult to achieve. In England, the number of GPs reduced from 0.52 per 1,000 patients in 2015, to 0.44 per 1,000 patients in 2022.[19] There are fewer GPs working full time and more are leaving the profession, due to the pressures of the job and increasing workloads. This means appointments are shorter and it's harder to see the same doctor every time, which in turn reduces the opportunities to develop good doctor–patient relationships.

Before qualifying, my impression from TV programmes, films and books was that a doctor's job was to make a diagnosis and treat the patient. In my first year of medical practice, the popular US drama *House* started to be broadcast. Its lead, Dr Gregory House, was played by English actor Hugh Laurie, previously known for his comedic performances. This role was very different – Dr House was portrayed as being a brilliant diagnostician, solving the mystery of what condition the patient suffered from when other doctors had failed. This was always in time to save the patient's life and conveniently before the end of each episode. However, his bedside manner left a lot to be desired, and his communication with his patients and his colleagues was frequently lacking in empathy and emotion. While he does ultimately cure the patient (which is clearly crucial!) the way in which he does so may not suit everyone.

House demonstrates well the transactional model of medicine, where people come with something that is 'broken' and we 'fix' it. Although never named, this model was reinforced in medical school as being what medicine was about. We were encouraged to weigh all of the evidence in front of us collected from the patient's history, examination, investigations and then either make the diagnosis and treat it, or refer for further tests or specialist care. There was less about looking after patients over their lifespan and more about these individual encounters. Some medical specialities are more transactional in nature as doctors may only see a patient for a single episode of illness. An example is surgery, where once the patient has recovered from the procedure, they may not need to meet their surgeon again. Surgeons often say that a sign of successful treatment is when the patients don't come back. Transactional medicine is effective and efficient, but is it enough? For many patients, the answer is probably 'yes': they just want to be well and go back to their normal lives. But other people who have multiple conditions, or whose symptoms don't point to an obvious diagnosis, may need more complex care over a period of time.

The longer I've been a doctor, the more I understand the importance of another model of medicine, one that is more relationship-based, like the roles John Sassall and Rowena Christmas so clearly convey. Dr Helen Salisbury, a GP writing in the *British Medical Journal*, describes this as being care that 'focuses on the interaction between patient and doctor. Although the medical activity may be similar, there's another dimension to consider, which is the quality of that interaction.' She describes how over time as they get to know each other, the relationship develops and builds trust. This in itself creates efficiency, as the patient and doctor are better able to understand each other and so, unnecessary tests and referrals are avoided.[20] Again, some medical specialities are more suited to this model, such as general practice, where a patient and doctor may know each other for decades. An integral part of the relationship-based model of care is continuity – seeing the same doctor every time, who is familiar with you and your life story. This is something that is increasingly uncommon, despite evidence that it improves the long-term health of patients.

This distinction between transactional and relationship-based models of care raises several questions:

What *is* the role of a doctor?

Are doctors merely 'fixers' like mechanics, or are they something more – such as 'healers'?

What happens when doctors are unable to 'fix' a patient – do they still hold any worth to society? This existential threat to our own value is an important driver of why we doctors find it difficult to listen.

Not knowing what ails a patient, nor how to treat them, is a surprisingly common situation for doctors. Patients with symptoms that are not medically explained make up 15–30 per cent of consultations in general practice in England.[21] Often these are self-limiting and the symptoms clear up by themselves over time. For example, this could be a nagging pain in the abdomen, which comes and goes and then disappears after a week. However, many unexplained symptoms persist. For patients, the consequences of not getting a diagnosis may be profound. A diagnosis means you know what's wrong with you and what to expect. You know that other people have had your illness and you are not alone in this. It can be a relief to get a diagnosis, so not getting one can feel incredibly disheartening.

This can be challenging for doctors, who have to manage this uncertainty. These are the situations where we are often at our most paternalistic and when we label patients as being 'difficult'. Before we had effective treatments, a doctor's role was to relieve suffering, not to cure disease or prevent death. With treatment advances in the twentieth century, this has changed and considerable investment has been devoted to medical research focused on reversing the main causes of death, such as cardiovascular disease and infectious diseases. This has meant that conditions that are less life-threatening, but still a significant cause of suffering, have been given a lower priority.[22] We do not know how to treat these conditions and sometimes we may not know what to do with symptoms we cannot explain.

Doctors have limitations, but sometimes we do not fully acknowledge them to our patients or even ourselves. This means patients may believe doctors have greater powers than they actually do, and doctors may believe in their own hubris. Not knowing is scary and makes us question our abilities. People who enter the caring professions are often those that want to help, to solve problems and make people better. They are natural 'fixers'. If we can't fix a patient, what is the point of us? This worry makes it harder for us to listen and we may close down conversations, or dismiss patients who make us question our sense of self. We don't recognise that patients may want us to tell them about our uncertainty. In fact, research shows that patients understand that doctors are fallible – they would prefer that we were more honest about diagnostic uncertainty, so that together we could come up with a realistic plan of action.[23] This may increase their trust in their doctor, and help them to make an informed decision about what to do next.

One of the most common conditions that doctors find difficult to 'fix' is chronic pain. This is defined as pain lasting for more than three months. It can have a devastating impact on people's lives and on how they see themselves. The British journalist Kirsty Young described in an interview how she had to step away from her work for several years after developing chronic pain due to rheumatoid arthritis and fibromyalgia.[24] She said of her experiences, 'It grinds you away, you lose your personality, you lose your sense of humour, you lose your sense of self.' Chronic pain is a complex and often misunderstood condition.[25] Individuals experience pain in different ways and this is affected by different biological and psychological factors and social situations. Pain is isolating, exhausting and wears people down. Experts in pain agree that it needs a multi-pronged approach that goes beyond just medication.

Consultations between doctors and people living with chronic pain may be fraught, with both finding them uncomfortable and unsatisfactory. Dr Jonathon Tomlinson, a GP working in a deprived area of inner London, has written thoughtfully about this, after noticing that many of his consultations were related to chronic pain. He found that patients with chronic pain were contacting the surgery three times more commonly than the average, at about thirty-three times a year. This was more than every fortnight – highlighting their elevated needs for healthcare.[26] Prompted by a frustrating consultation he'd had with such a patient, Tomlinson wrote a blog asking 'Why then is it so hard for doctors and patients to cope with chronic pain?'[27] He describes seeing a patient known to him to discuss her pain. The discussion went badly and ended up with her accusing him of not doing anything for her: 'You don't even know what's wrong with me and now you're trying to tell me it's all in my head, you're not listening to me!' Tomlinson was hurt by this, feeling that over the years he'd actually done a lot – referring her to different specialists and supporting her and her family through difficult times in their lives. However, clearly it had not been enough and he concluded that he had nothing left to offer. He realised that it wasn't that he hadn't been listening, it was that he had been listening *in the wrong way*. 'I had failed to acknowledge her suffering and she didn't believe that I believed her.'

He understood the suffering to include the onerous task of having to explain her symptoms again and again to healthcare professionals and her friends and family. People with chronic pain often describe the isolation and alienation they feel from their loved ones, their doctors and even from their own bodies. Novelist Sarah Perry, writing of her own painful illness, said that, 'The problem with describing pain, of course, is that you can no more know what I mean by torment than I can know what you mean by love – and besides, privately we all think ourselves made of sterner stuff than the sickly.'[28] This difficulty in communication, coupled with the shame that she describes, is one of the reasons for this loneliness. Chronic pain is not glamorous or dramatic and does not garner the same amount of sympathy that other conditions like a heart attack or cancer may get. It means that it causes a type of suffering that is invisible and unwitnessed.

For doctors, we find consultations with patients experiencing chronic pain difficult because we feel we cannot help them. Reaching a point where you feel that you have nothing more to offer a patient can be devastating, making us feel like we are failures. We may also feel responsible for their pain, which makes us even less open to hearing about it. So, we avoid these conversations, creating diversions such as offering questionnaires to measure their pain (please score your pain between 1–10), refer the patient to other healthcare professionals or offer another prescription for painkillers that are often ineffectual. All of these actions make us feel like we are doing something, but these diversions can lead to over-investigation and unnecessary treatment, which in itself can be harmful. We prefer to see patients we feel we can treat. Patients we can't treat are 'difficult'.

What if doctors took a different approach? What if we just listened, letting the patient tell us about the nature of their suffering? Would this act of bearing witness and validation not be in itself healing? We know that patients find value in this. However, this is not incentivised in modern medicine – funding is often based on *doing* something, be that a blood test or making a diagnosis and treating it. Listening and bearing witness is not as easy to measure, is not viewed as being productive and is not valued in the same way. It may also go against our instincts to 'do nothing'. In her essay 'The art of doing nothing', Dr Iona Heath argues that in contrast, this apparent 'doing nothing' can be an active and deliberate process.[29] Listening closely without interrupting, and hearing things that make us feel uncomfortable, is hard work. Bearing witness is also an active process. By doing this, you are offering companionship and telling a person that you are there *with* them, in solidarity. GPs are good at this – trained to know when to reassure patients, to hold uncertainty about diagnosis and to recognise when to refer onwards.

In his now classic 1982 paper and subsequent book *The Nature of Suffering and the Goals of Medicine*, medical ethicist Eric Cassell wrote of suffering as being more than just physical pain, but something that affects the whole person.[30] He challenged doctors to recognise that 'the relief of suffering and the cure of disease must be seen as twin obligations of a medical profession that is truly dedicated to the care of the sick'. He argued that by not understanding this, doctors failed to not only relieve their patient's suffering, but exacerbated it. This goes back to rethinking what the role of a doctor actually is. If we were to regard ourselves as healers rather than just fixers, then we would see more value in listening. The relationship-based model of care encourages this, but we need to ensure that opportunities to strengthen the doctor–patient relationship do not disappear. Currently it is under threat, but I want to show you how valuable it can be.

*

'Doctor, you won't believe it, but James is putting in his application for medical school! He asked me to tell you.' Linda grinned as she updated me on the latest news about her oldest son.

I had first met Linda fifteen years earlier when she was admitted to our hospital for several months. Diagnosed with advanced HIV, she needed treatment for multiple infections and had almost died. That was my first year as an HIV doctor and I spent half of it on the ward, learning how to treat the sickest of patients with AIDS-related conditions. Linda and I were of a similar age and got to know each other over that time. She was a single mum and her sister used to bring James, a toddler at the time, to visit.

Years later when I came back to the department as a consultant, I was delighted to meet her again in clinic. We caught up on the intervening time, and I found that with the help of HIV anti-retroviral therapy, she was healthy and doing well. She had married again and had qualified as a solicitor.

'That's great news! Doesn't time fly? I can still remember when he was little, coming in to see you in hospital. That smile! We'd all be fighting over who could give him some of the ward chocolate just to see it!' I laughed.

'I know . . . and look at him now – wanting to work in a hospital himself. I'm so proud.'

'You must be! Please congratulate him for me.' I clasped her hand. 'So what about you – how are you doing? Did you get your back looked at by the physio?' I asked.

'I did . . . but you know what my work is like. I'm always at my desk on the computer, or having meetings. It just makes it worse . . .' We continued the consultation and I booked to see her in six months' time.

This is an example of a doctor–patient relationship that has been developed over a period of time. There is a sense of familiarity and trust – we are partners in Linda's care and know how to communicate with each other. We don't need to start from scratch, which saves time and as efficiency is often the counter-argument to this approach, it's important to highlight this. As an HIV doctor, I feel fortunate to have this continuity of care, knowing some of my patients for more than fifteen years, or since their first positive HIV test. As the years go on, we gather knowledge about each other and this is good for both of us.

The British Medical Association says that the doctor–patient relationship is 'critical to good person-centred health'. It describes four key principles to this relationship:[31]

1. Both doctors and patients have obligations to treat each other with honesty and respect, but doctors have particular duties to patients which are rooted in their professional status.
2. Doctors must make the care of patients their first concern.
3. For good communication, both sides need to be open, honest and to listen.
4. Good patient care must take into account the patient as a whole person.

This shows how the doctor–patient relationship relies on both parties being willing to make it work. Researchers have found that the depth of the relationship depends on knowledge, trust, loyalty and regard, seen from both the patient's perspective about the doctor, and vice versa.[32] A study of people who saw the same family doctor for more than fifteen years found that they chose to do so because the doctor already had some knowledge of them, they were familiar with the doctor, confident in their expertise and satisfied with the care they received. They also found they had developed a friendship and found it easy to communicate.[33]

The doctor–patient relationship is not just beneficial for patients. It is also a source of joy and job satisfaction for doctors. To know people over years and to be with them during the ups and downs of their lives, is meaningful and sustains us. In my own experience, and Sassall's and Christmas', these are the stories that fulfil us and make the profession more satisfying. Beyond this, there is plenty of evidence that continuity of care is good for patients. Patients who have seen the same family doctor for a year or longer, are a quarter less likely to use emergency services.[34] You may have noticed it yourself, feeling more able to share how you're really feeling with a doctor if you've met them before and had a good experience. Certainly, as a doctor, I often find that it's a relief to see someone I'm familiar with as I'm not starting from scratch, but already know their background.

However, not all patients want to have a relationship-based model of care with their doctor. They may prefer more transactional care, or to see the first doctor available in the most convenient location for them. This means it is really important to provide a choice of appointments.

Despite continuity of care being described as an essential feature of general practice, it is under threat. This is due to services becoming more fragmented, a changing workforce with changing work patterns (more doctors working less than full time) and an emphasis on rapid access (seeing the first doctor available, not necessarily your doctor).[35] This means that patients often need to take the initiative to maintain continuity of care. But this is not always easy – they may have to navigate confusing telephone and computer systems to book the appointment with the doctor they want. This is more difficult for some groups of patients, particularly the elderly, those with mental health conditions and the socially vulnerable. Ironically these are the people who are most likely to benefit from seeing the same doctor. Healthcare services can support continuity of care too, by making appointment systems easier to use and anticipating which patients may need help with booking. They can also offer a range of appointments which mean that patients can be seen quickly if ill, or can book a few weeks ahead if it's not urgent and they want to see a particular doctor.

The doctor–patient relationship can be very powerful. It requires a mutual willing to trust and respect each other, and both sides have their responsibilities. For doctors, these are related in their codes of professional practice such as their duty of care to the patient. When it's working well, it can have a huge beneficial impact on the patient's health, as well as providing the doctor with a sense of job satisfaction. However, there are several important ethical issues that are relevant with regards to the relationship, including patient autonomy so that they are able to make their own decisions about their care, and the maintenance of professional boundaries. These boundaries acknowledge the power imbalance between the patient and the doctor and are there to protect both. For example, doctors must not enter into a sexual relationship with a patient; they should avoid treating a family member; they should decline large gifts. These are obvious examples of boundaries, but there are others which are less defined and are related to communication. These work at an individual and systematic level and can affect how much patients are heard. If we could build an understanding of these into medical training it could help us better fulfil our role without overextending ourselves emotionally and burning out in the process.

*

They trudged off the ward in silence, heads down. As they waited for the lift to take them to the next stop on the ward round, Ashley, the most junior doctor in the team, gave a big sigh. Picking up on this, the consultant asked him if he was all right.

'I'm OK thanks. It's just . . . it's just that I always feel really drained after seeing Mrs Drew on the round.'

The other two junior doctors in the team nodded in agreement, adding, 'I know what you mean. She's exhausting.' And, 'She's so angry, but why does she have to take it out on us? It's not our fault. We're just trying to do our best for her. I've started to dread visiting her every day.'

Mrs Drew had been admitted to hospital three months earlier with fever and pain after recent routine knee replacement surgery. She'd developed a serious post-operative infection and needed to have more surgery and intravenous antibiotics. After weeks in intensive care, she was stepped down to the surgical ward. Despite physiotherapy, her recovery was slow and she was awaiting a bed in a nearby rehabilitation facility to get her stronger before she could go home. Before this admission, she'd been an active member of the local church community and volunteered at the library, her energy belying her seventy years.

Now stuck in hospital and mostly confined to her bed, she was no longer able to keep up her good humour, so desperate was she to go home. She regularly took out her frustration on the staff looking after her. This morning had been particularly difficult as she realised she would still be in hospital for her grandson's eighteenth birthday, and would miss the celebration. During the ward round, she furiously accused her doctors of deliberately keeping her in and stopping her from seeing him. It was an uncomfortable experience for all present.

The consultant looked at her team and said, 'If that's how she makes you feel after seeing her, imagine feeling like that all the time, like she does. What you are experiencing is her anger and frustration about being so ill for so long, with no hope of getting home soon. At least for you, these emotions are only temporary – she can't escape hers, and her way of coping is to share it with us. But I get how bad you are feeling... I feel it too. It's draining. It's good to talk about this.'

Her team looked relieved at her admission and the conversation continued over coffee after the ward round.

The consultant had done her team a great service in this scenario – she had introduced them to the concept of 'transference'. This was coined by Sigmund Freud and describes what happens when a person projects their emotions onto another individual.[36] This can commonly happen in psychotherapy and caring professions. By talking to her team about this, the consultant normalised how they were feeling. She reminded them to put themselves in the position of the patient who was having a terrible time and to maintain their empathy for her. She also acknowledged that such conversations are common and prepared them for the inevitability of similar encounters in the future.

Listening to stories of suffering on a daily basis can be exhausting. This is because they can trigger in the listener emotions like overidentification, grief, trauma, self-sacrifice and guilt. Maintaining some separation from the patient is important for doctors. This distancing has other purposes – it helps doctors to be objective about a patient's predicament in a way that perhaps the patient cannot be. Boundaries also protect patients from 'counter-transference' where the practitioner projects their own emotions onto their patient. But listening is a fundamental part of medicine and doctors need to learn to cope with it when it becomes uncomfortable, and to not let it affect their interactions with patients. There is a fine line between maintaining boundaries and being fully present with patients. Medical students are taught to consider their individual approach to balancing listening well with maintaining professional detachment.

In his essay 'Emotions are Contagious', GP Jonathon Tomlinson describes how doctors and patients communicate in ways that they may not even be aware of.[37] Without realising, they pick up on each other's emotions. If a doctor feels uncomfortable with what the patient is saying (verbally or non-verbally), the patient picks up on this unease and may feel further distressed. This ramps up the tension further, making the consultation increasingly difficult and potentially adversarial. Patients who have experienced different forms of trauma in their lives are more sensitised to any form of potential threat. These are the patients who are more likely to pick up on their doctor's unease, possibly before they do, and their innate defensive responses kick in faster. Tomlinson argues that by learning to better tolerate distress, doctors will become not only better at listening, but at listening in a way that is therapeutic for the patient. By being present, by appearing centred and calm, we can relieve a patient's suffering. This is not easy and requires self-reflection and practice. Tomlinson recommends different methods to try and increase tolerance to distress. For example, he has tried the Wim Hof method of cold exposure, standing in a freezing cold shower to improve his tolerance. Such methods may not suit all doctors (including me!) but I think that by practising listening without interruption or diversion, we can learn to do this. I liken this to developing a listening muscle – one that makes us better able to cope with the work of witnessing suffering.

While boundaries are learnt and practised by individuals, they can also become institutionalised, integrated in healthcare service policies and protocols. The danger here is that they may go too far, taking the humanity out of the care system, which is damaging for patients and healthcare workers. This was shown clearly in a 1960 research paper, its findings still valid today.[38] The author, psychologist Isabel Menzies, was asked to investigate why a third of the nursing students at a large London teaching hospital had dropped out of their training programme. The students expressed to her high levels of anxiety due to both the close contact they had with patients and the responsibility of caring for them. Menzies found that the hospital had introduced multiple strategies over time to cope with this stress. These included diluting the nurse–patient relationship by giving each nurse fewer tasks to perform on an increased number of patients. This prevented them from spending too much time with a particular patient and getting too close. Rituals, flow charts and guidelines had been introduced to take away the stress of making decisions. Hospital culture encouraged staff to maintain a 'stiff upper lip', detaching them from their emotions. Menzies also noticed that the use of dehumanising language was widespread, such as referring to an individual as 'the pneumonia in bed fifteen'. Menzies described these as 'socially structured defence mechanisms' which she felt were core to how the institution operated. Despite being designed to alleviate nurses' anxiety, they actually made it worse. They took out the 'whole person aspect' of care, creating automation and reducing the nurses' sense of personal accomplishment and development. By taking much of the risk out of the job for individual nurses, they took out much of the satisfaction. The defence mechanisms also reduced opportunities to learn how to better cope in stressful situations.

Although this study is over sixty years old it is still relevant, showing how services can be too risk-averse, creating professional boundaries that are too rigid and bad for healthcare workers and patients. There are policies that can help healthcare workers better cope with close patient contact. These include self-reflection, debriefing with colleagues, mentoring and supervision. This already exists in some caring professions. For example, in psychotherapy, practitioners are required to have supervision, which is an opportunity to talk about the emotional impact of patient care in a confidential and safe space. In hospital teams, this is something that happens ad hoc after a traumatic event such as an unexpected patient death, or in the scenario of transference that I have described. However, the opportunities for debriefing could be widened, integrating the practice into training and working lives. Formal mentoring may be a solution, employing senior doctors who are coming to the end of their careers. By this point, they have built up a vast bank of expertise after decades of interacting with patients, so may be ideal candidates to mentor others. Schemes also exist to incorporate peer supervision. For example, clinician and educator John Launer has, over several decades, run courses in Conversations Inviting Change. This invites doctors to discuss and reflect on cases with their peers.[39] It teaches narrative-based medicine, which recognises that everyone has a need to tell stories and looks at how this may be used therapeutically for patients and doctors. These examples are all methods which could systematically improve patient experience by better equipping doctors to listen, while maintaining professional boundaries. Certainly, I find debriefing with colleagues after a challenging encounter helpful – it's a chance to talk about how I am feeling, and to learn from them. These methods may also protect doctors who are vulnerable to developing compassion fatigue and burnout.

I first became aware of the term 'compassion fatigue' during the second year of the COVID-19 pandemic, when our departmental psychology team held a session on it for staff. Working in a large sexual health and HIV centre, we are fortunate to have an inhouse psychology team to support patients with their mental health. During the pandemic, when many staff were redeployed to COVID-19 wards, our psychologists kindly redirected their efforts to supporting the mental health of their colleagues. They provided drop-in sessions and confidential spaces where we could talk about how we were feeling. Compassion fatigue is characterised by the mental, physical and emotional exhaustion resulting from caring for individuals enduring trauma or suffering. During the COVID-19 pandemic, healthcare staff were seeing more suffering than ever. This, combined with the moral injury of not being able to practice the best care possible due to the lack of resources, was leading to widespread compassion fatigue.[40] This meant that staff who were feeling drained had fewer internal resources to provide the standard of care they normally did to patients. They were less able to listen and show compassion.

Compassion fatigue can be a precursor to burnout, a more

complete exhaustion which is not only related to the work of caring, but all aspects of work. It has been found to be particularly common among healthcare workers globally and significantly impacts patient care. A large review of research studies found that doctors with burnout were twice as likely to have been involved in patient safety incidents, to be rated poorly by their patients on their quality of care and to show lower levels of professionalism. Doctors became cynical, negative, callous and had a more detached attitude to their work. Burnt-out doctors were four times more likely to be dissatisfied with their job, three times more likely to regret their choice of career and three times more likely to want to leave the profession.[41]

Doctor wellbeing is a patient safety issue. When doctors experience compassion fatigue or burnout, they are less able to treat patients with empathy and to fully hear them. They make mistakes which can lead to misdiagnosis, neglect and maltreatment. They increase patient suffering. By preventing compassion fatigue and burnout, doctors are less likely to leave, improving the quality and safety of patient care. Since the COVID-19 pandemic in particular, health organisations have introduced schemes offering staff psychological support. However, when resources are stretched, and staff are working harder than ever for increasing numbers of patients, it is vital that staff wellbeing includes safe workplaces with fair remuneration. This requires politicians to listen to healthcare staff. It is more urgent than ever that we take steps to protect doctors and other healthcare professionals, and give them the tools they need to form healthy boundaries, and care for themselves. With this shift we could work towards fairer and more equal interactions.

*

The act of listening is of vital importance in medicine, where people are at their most vulnerable. Without hearing what a patient is saying, a doctor cannot understand their needs, make a diagnosis, treat them or comfort them. A conversation is a dynamic process between the speaker and the listener. The listener is equally as important as the speaker, as their response encourages or inhibits how much and what the speaker will say. For example, if the speaker sees that the listener is angered, disgusted or dismissive of what they say, they may decide that it is not safe to continue, so they stop speaking – they are silenced. The listener must convey curiosity, be non-judgemental and be prepared to not give advice. Doctors also learn more about a patient from careful listening, as we start to take notice of what they are conveying through their body language and behaviour.

Many research studies have looked at what behaviours encourage better conversations between family doctors and patients, and consequently better health outcomes.[42] These included a doctor showing empathy and courtesy, reassurance, making questions more 'patient-centred', giving time, positive reinforcement, using humour at the appropriate time, providing explanations, summarising and clarifying. Non-verbal cues included leaning forwards, nodding, uncrossing arms and legs.

Body language is important and something we were taught at medical school – how to sit with an open stance to encourage confidences, mirroring someone's movements, avoiding defensive postures like crossing our arms. Sitting next to a person and not giving them direct eye contact may make them feel less pressured, and so encouraged to talk. When I was training, one of my consultants taught me to be on the same level as patients in their beds. I still do this, grabbing a chair to speak to a patient sitting in bed, or squatting so that my eyes are on the same level as a patient lying down. When you are unwell in hospital, having a group of doctors towering over you from the end of the bed reinforces your feeling of powerlessness – having things done *to* you, rather than in consultation *with* you. Another way of reducing this power imbalance is by giving patients choices about where and when to talk.

I really got to understand the importance of verbal and non-verbal communication during the start of the COVID-19 pandemic, where wearing personal protective equipment such as masks and visors created a distance with patients. I had to concentrate harder on what I said, adjust my tone, and try to show comfort in different ways – a touch on a shoulder, holding a hand instead of smiling.

Individual doctors have their own methods of encouraging people to talk, some more successful than others.

One that I have picked up is 'code-switching'. This involves an individual changing their style of speech, expression and behaviour in order to increase the comfort of others. This has been discussed widely in recent years, with people of colour describing how they may do this to fit in with white cultural norms. If a person feels forced to code-switch, this may be harmful to them, particularly if this is required to fit in with workplace culture. I have been code-switching most of my life, sometimes without even noticing. I will never forget my astonishment when my husband, visiting India with me for the first time, pointed out that I changed my accent, the speed and the rhythm of my speech when I spoke with my relatives. This made it easier for them to understand me, but I had never done it deliberately. At work, I sometimes code-switch with patients. As a sexual health doctor, I have to encourage my patients to share the most intimate aspects of their lives with me. I will adjust my language and the way in which I speak depending on, for example, the age of the patient. Older patients may prefer their doctors to be more formal, whereas younger ones may feel more comfortable with informality. When code-switching is done intentionally and with care, it can be very useful. But it must be done without stereotyping people and understanding that each person is an individual. I once worked in a sexual health clinic in Essex and found my teenage accent returning when having a consultation with a young person. I'm not sure the patient noticed, but for me, it felt a step too far and I was worried I was coming across as patronising.

I also have some practical strategies for consultations that work for me. These include writing down key bits of information and useful websites for patients, and giving leaflets, so they have something to take away with them. I try to make my language as simple and clear as I can, and I regularly pause to check they understand me. Before they leave, I will summarise any next steps and try and manage their expectations as to when things will happen. For example, 'I have booked a scan, but this may not happen for a couple of weeks.' If I am concerned a patient has not taken everything in, I will offer them a chance to bring someone with them next time. If we run out of time, I will organise a follow-up appointment.

Palliative care doctor Kathryn Mannix says in her book *Listen* that, 'Listening is a skill we can learn. Many of us learn it by trial and error, mistake and reflection. Perhaps it is a skill to include in the transmission of wisdom down the generations. It may even have its place in school curricula.'[43] When I left medical school twenty years ago, I had comprehensive knowledge of the body, including how it worked, what happened when it became ill and how to manage this. I had the skills to diagnose and treat disease, but I left without knowing how to treat *people*. It could be argued that these are skills that can't be taught but come with years of experience at the coalface – I improved my listening through such experience and practice. However, I also believe it would have been useful to know how 'to practice medicine in an imperfect world' earlier in my learning; to anticipate that some patients require relationship-based care, while others prefer transactional care; to understand the limitations of medicine and to know what to do with uncertainty; to learn the origins of stereotypes and how bias affects medical practice. It would have been useful to know how the wider social determinants of health affect people and how they are able to engage in healthy behaviours. To some degree, I think I have spent much of my working life 'unlearning' medical school.

I acknowledge it may be different today, and so I spoke with Riya George, reader in Clinical Communication Skills and Diversity Education at Barts and The London School of Medicine and Dentistry, to find out how. She told me that clinical communication skills are highly prioritised, with teaching starting in Year 1. Students now get an opportunity to take part in practice OSCES, where they can receive feedback without their marks having future consequences. There have also been efforts to promote more person-centred care; for example, encouraging students to avoid depersonalising language. Over Zoom, I asked her what she thought could be done to improve clinical communication skills training. She replied, 'The one thing would be inviting patients, and not in a tokenistic way of just hearing their story, but in how we develop the curriculum and how we design it.' She pointed out the 'baffling' paradox of teaching medical students how to talk to patients, yet not having patients involved. This seems a really important point to me and makes clear to students the notion that patients can be equal partners with doctors right from the start of training. After graduation, doctors should also be assessed regularly on their communication skills. This happens to an extent in the UK where all doctors go through a revalidation process every five years to ensure they are fit to practice.[44] As part of this, we must provide patient feedback. We ask a series of consecutive patients to fill out an anonymous survey so they can rate us on different aspects of our care. This includes whether they were listened to and how we made them feel. While it is possible to influence the results by only giving the survey to patients you know you have a good relationship with, this can still be a useful measure if done properly. We are also asked to provide evidence of feedback from a wide range of colleagues who anonymously assess us on our performance.

I have learnt that in order to listen well as a doctor we must: 1) hear what the patient is saying and not saying, 2) hear what their body language is telling us and 3) hear what our own body is telling us in response to them. At the core of this is knowing ourselves – our triggers, our blind spots and biases, how we respond to different types of patient and information. For me this is a variation on the biblical proverb 'Physician, heal thyself', to 'Physician, hear thyself', and is crucial to ensure we listen better. Through regular reflection and feedback from both patients and colleagues, we can work to improve our listening skills throughout our careers. I believe that this can also be enhanced through an increased appreciation that medicine is an art as well as being a science.

Because there is real art to medicine. It requires skill and knowledge and is based in human values and intuition. I believe the arts have made me a better doctor and researcher. Through fiction I learnt of other worlds and how people I would never meet lived. Through visual art, I felt a sense of being small, but part of something greater and more beautiful than I could imagine. They grounded me and continue to do so. I still read fiction every day to relax, and can be found carefully placing blobs of acrylic paint on canvas if the time and space allows. These are components of my life outside of work that keep me going. They deliver psychological and even spiritual sustenance at times and provide an important counterfoil to the often emotionally draining aspects of my work. At university, I became an active member of the student union's art society and undertook a study module on the history of medicine, writing my thesis on childbirth through the ages. For the first time, I was introduced to how women have experienced sexism in healthcare, which was eye-opening and not taught in the main curriculum, where the emphasis was on science. In my research career, I have been fortunate to work with medical philosophers, sociologists and historians, collaborations which I have found both fruitful and enjoyable. These projects have also helped me think about my clinical practice from different perspectives, which I feel has only enhanced it. This book is a culmination of these interests, and it has been a joy to research a range of topics from such different fields on top of more conventional scientific texts.

Many people are calling for the greater involvement of the medical humanities in the student curriculum. These include philosophy of medicine, ethics, bioethics, history of medicine, narrative medicine, religion, medical anthropology, sociology, literature, film, visual arts and theatre. The medical humanities use interdisciplinary research to explore the experiences of health and illness. If medicine is viewed to be an art as well as a science, then an understanding of the medical humanities may complement the more scientific aspects of the curriculum. The General Medical Council recommend that doctors understand a patient's psychological, social and cultural needs alongside their pathology.[45] By including humanities in the medical curriculum, they may help doctors develop a deeper understanding of patients' illness journeys, reducing paternalism, increasing empathy and patient-focused care. They will have a better understanding of the individuals and communities they serve. The humanities may also improve doctors' interpersonal skills with colleagues and provide an outlet when stressed.

Dr Giskin Day teaches medical humanities at the School of Medicine at Imperial College London and is passionate about how the medical humanities complement and enrich clinical teaching. She gave the example of locked-in syndrome, a rare condition where patients are paralysed, but conscious and only able to communicate by blinking. Students may learn about the pathology behind this in their neurology placements, but by reading Jean-Dominique Bauby's novel *The Diving-bell and the Butterfly*, they develop a deeper insight into what it is like to live with it. Her hope is that students feel that they are capable of being creative and that this will help them in their future careers to come up with innovative solutions to problems. Day told me about the different ways in which sessions are facilitated to stimulate conversations – from visiting art galleries to reading poetry and novels. Students can create their own pieces of art. As I spoke to her, I wished that I had access to such a course when I was at university. The worlds of art and science are intrinsically linked, as imperfect and multifaceted as the humans they stem from. Day told me how having cataracts affected Impressionist painter Claude Monet's vision, and consequently his work. His condition transformed the colour scheme of his paintings from cool blues and greens to warm yellows, oranges and reds. As his eyesight became more blurred, his brush strokes become wider. He put off cataract surgery for many years, and this is brilliantly depicted in the poem 'Monet Refuses the Operation' by Lisel Mueller.[46] In Day's teaching sessions, students visit Monet's paintings and are invited to write their own poem in the form of a letter to Monet in response to his decision. Why is this important? Well, it shows how patients make decisions that we as doctors may not initially understand (why wouldn't Monet want his eyesight improved?) and how their motivations may differ from ours. Perhaps Monet's view of the world worked for him.

Medical humanities prepare doctors to treat people, not just diseases. And an important part of this is listening and paying attention to their narratives. If more doctors are exposed to arts and the medical humanities, it may widen perspectives and encourage humility when interacting with patients and each other. Without the humanities, I certainly would not have felt capable or creative enough to write this book.

*

When empathy and openness are missing from our healthcare system, we lose the fundamental core of why healthcare exists in the first place. We let the transactional displace the relational, and compassion and care are replaced with data and assumption. From the very start, in university, we are taught methods which favour a style of medicine that instils hubris, reinforces power structures and casts doubt on patients. We are in danger of losing the art of medicine, the human core that appreciates that forming firm relationships with patients is what makes the job so worth doing. The role of the doctor has transformed itself into one which can be harmful for doctors themselves, resulting in compassion fatigue, burnout and stress; it is one that can instil further injustice by not seeing patients as individuals, and lean too heavily into science and a belief that medicine is the perfect cure for all ailments.

Between planning this book and writing it, I returned to clinical work after a year away studying for a master's degree. This was the first time I had taken a break longer than a month since qualifying as a doctor seventeen years previously. While studying stretched me intellectually, time away from hospital gave me some head space which I needed after working through the first two years of the COVID-19 pandemic. I'm grateful to my colleagues and employers for allowing me this time. Coming back to patient care, my intention was to be a better listener, making myself present in consultations to ensure my patients felt heard. This has not been easy, however much I tried. I have found myself reflecting daily on what has gone well and what hasn't. Stepping back onto the treadmill, I now appreciate that being a doctor is tough – it can be gruelling trying to do your best within a system that often works against you. But listening is fundamental to good medicine. Unless we do it well, patients suffer and can even die. We see this in patient safety reports all the time. When we don't listen to patients, we don't treat them as partners in their care and this can make them withdraw, silencing them. I'm not arguing that listening to patients means always doing what they request. A vital part of a doctor's role is to be a patient's advocate, which includes acting in a patient's best interests. If a request is unnecessary or harmful, then a doctor has the right to refuse it, but should explain why, and ensure the patient is aware that they can get a second opinion. We must however make sure the patient feels that their request and the reasons for it have been heard.

Listening can be beautiful, with real depth of understanding and affinity achieved in those quiet moments of connection with patients and colleagues. We don't often get the time to just stop and acknowledge this, but I feel lucky to have had the opportunity to do so. When I asked Jonathon Tomlinson what we can do to listen better, he replied, 'We need to be more open-hearted.' Patients deserve to feel that, when they are at their most vulnerable, they can be met with the same openness.

Summary: How doctors can listen better

- Training doctors at medical school:
  - Include patients in designing the curriculum.
  - Share some sessions with students from the allied health professions.
  - Training on how to listen well, and the importance of it.
  - Give opportunities to discuss and reflect on practicing medicine in the real world with the non-ideal patient. Include scenarios on uncomfortable conversations including dealing with uncertainty.
  - Teach about the social determinants of health, health equity and bias.
  - Offer opportunities to study the medical humanities.

- For individuals:
  - Reflect on your own listening practice – when is listening hard? How do you know when you need a break? What are your blind spots and potential biases? What can you do to be more prepared for uncomfortable conversations?
  - Think about how you can be more curious and open when listening. How can you listen with less judgement? Is it possible that the patient's point is valid, even if you don't necessarily agree with it?
  - How can you make patients feel heard, and reassured that what they say is important to you?
  - Find opportunities to debrief with colleagues.

- For managers in healthcare settings:
  - Create listening environments such as dedicated private spaces for conversations.
  - Build in short breaks to clinical sessions. Lengthen the time available for consultations if required.
  - Implement regular supervision and mentoring schemes.

- o Consider ways to reduce individual bias through protocols.
- o Provide staff with wellbeing services such as counselling, access to food and drinks, rest spaces.
- o Provide safe spaces for staff to be listened to, and act on concerns.

- For policymakers:
  - o Introduce policies that promote continuity of care and patient choice about appointments.
  - o Look at how listening can be incentivised through measurements assessing patient experience.
  - o Ensure listening and communication continues to be a priority in ongoing doctor education and assessment throughout the course of a career.

3

Excluded

When Doctors Aren't Heard

My first response was outrage.

And then I started to doubt myself.

It was late spring 2020 and media outlets were starting to report that people from Black, Asian and other ethnic minority communities in the UK were being disproportionately affected by COVID-19. In comparison to white communities, they were more likely to be admitted to hospital and to need intensive care. They were more likely to die. I had begun to notice this in my clinical practice too. These were the people I had been seeing on the wards as I'd carried out my rounds, their frightened faces struggling for breath behind see-through oxygen masks, made cloudy with COVID-19 secretions. Seeing so many patients who looked like me and my relatives was a bewildering experience and I remember feeling constantly dissatisfied with myself. Whatever I had done that day at work, I came home feeling that it wasn't enough – the emotional tidal wave of the global pandemic had left me with the recurrent thought, *Is there more I can do?*

In the absence of research evidence pointing to the causes of this disparity, speculation was rife on medical Twitter. Was it a genetic issue? Was it low vitamin D levels? Perhaps it was because Black and brown people had more underlying conditions like diabetes that made them more susceptible to COVID-19? I had spent several years researching racial inequity in health and was regularly invited to teach on the topic, so I felt I could usefully contribute to the conversation. I wanted to emphasise that in the UK, racial health inequalities were not new. They had existed well before COVID-19, were widespread throughout medicine, and had barely improved. They existed predominantly due to the effects of structural racism and social inequality, not culture or genetics as was being widely suggested.

I spent the morning of my day off preparing a meticulously researched and referenced Twitter thread of statistics. These showed racial inequalities in a wide range of health conditions. These included statistics such as, in comparison to white people in the UK:

- Black men are twice as likely to be diagnosed with prostate cancer and proportionately more likely to die of it.
- Black people are more likely to have asthma.
- South Asian and Black people are three to five times more likely to start kidney dialysis.
- South Asian and Black people are three to five times more likely to be diagnosed with Type 2 diabetes.

My hope was that it would demonstrate clearly how the health of racially minoritised communities had been historically under-prioritised. I wanted to galvanise people into action! I pressed the 'send tweet' button and prepared myself for the response.

The first reply was not one I had anticipated. A man I hadn't interacted with before on Twitter said, 'Is this true and has it been medically fact checked?' I was taken aback, feeling this was an attack on the data I presented and my authority as the person presenting it. I was particularly puzzled as my Twitter biography had my title (Dr), job description (consultant physician) and place of work (a large teaching hospital).

'How dare he?!' I protested to my husband.

Then I started to wonder – what was it about me that made him say this? Did I lack credibility as a doctor? Did I come across as untrustworthy? Then the self-doubt started – perhaps I hadn't researched the thread thoroughly enough, perhaps I didn't know as much about the topic as I thought I did...

I realised these feelings of self-doubt were not new.

During my sixteen years and counting of being a doctor, I had felt the need to prove myself at work regularly, despite my growing qualifications and expertise. I suffered from impostor syndrome. This is defined as the persistent fear of being found out as a fraud, despite your accomplishments. It was first described in 1978 by psychology researchers Pauline R. Clance and Suzanne A. Imes as something they had observed among high-achieving career women. It has attracted much attention in recent years, particularly in medicine.[1,2]

On many occasions, I had been mistaken for a more junior colleague on the ward or had to repeat myself several times to get my view heard in meetings. I am a woman of Indian descent, scarcely five feet tall and I'm often told I 'have a nice smile'. I look younger than my years, something I'm sure I'll feel grateful for in the future. Nevertheless, in my profession this can be a liability as I am often under-estimated and discounted. Now working in the same team for many years, this experience is rare – my colleagues know me and respect my knowledge and skills. Only very occasionally, when I meet someone new or am in an unfamiliar area of the hospital, does this happen.

I realised early on in my career that as I didn't fit the stereotype of what a doctor looks like (white, male), it was important for me to take care with how I came across – always dressing and acting professionally, always prepared and making sure I knew everything about a patient's case or a topic before discussing it with colleagues. I understood that I couldn't get away with anything less than this level of performance. I became used to this – I was confident in my abilities, aware that my colleagues had the same confidence in me, but mindful that my authority could be doubted at any time by those unfamiliar with me.

I sensed a change at the start of the COVID-19 pandemic – my seniority was not being recognised again. Like many colleagues, I was keen to contribute to the pandemic effort – this was a global emergency and we wanted to do as much as we could. I was re-deployed from the HIV department to treat the influx of patients with COVID-19 in the first wave. I was apprehensive and, to be honest, a little scared. Even as an HIV doctor seasoned with treating some of the sickest patients in the hospital with infectious diseases, this was challenging – a new virus that we were learning more about every day; the worry that we would ourselves catch it and take it home to our loved ones. I knew of doctors who were updating their wills, just in case.

It was an unsettling time. A powerful memory that stays with me from those otherwise murky first days of March 2020 is of my colleagues disappearing on a daily basis – present in the HIV department one day, and not the next – be that from redeployment to COVID-19 wards, shielding at home or isolating due to their own illness or of someone in their household.

Redeployment to the COVID-19 wards meant being allocated to new teams on rotas with people I hadn't worked with before, often on unfamiliar wards. During a typical week on the rota, I would find myself leading a team of junior doctors, and these would change several times a week, depending on who had just done, or was about to do, a night shift. Working with a familiar face was always a source of delight – no introductions needed. For infection control purposes, we were all wearing scrubs. NHS scrubs at my hospital came in three standard sizes – all of them, on me, different degrees of 'billowing'. The smallest size still swamped me, making me look like a child trying on my parents' clothes. Gone was my professional 'work uniform' of sleek dresses and shiny shoes, all designed to help patients and colleagues have confidence in me. And, I realise, to instil confidence in myself.

I quickly came to understand that, on a daily basis, I was having to make an additional effort to assert my seniority. I'd be leading a COVID-19 round with my team when a visiting specialist team would come onto the ward to give an opinion about a patient. Invariably they'd start to talk to one of my junior white and male colleagues, assuming they were the ward consultant and in charge. I'd step forward, speaking louder than I normally would, to interrupt the conversation that had started without me. 'Hello, I'm Dr Rageshri, the consultant on the ward. How can we help you?' This always made me feel a little embarrassed and I think this feeling was shared by my team members and the visitors. Or I'd be questioned by a member of the ward staff about a prescription or paperwork that needed doing. They'd be forthright and often verging on rude in their request, until I introduced myself as the consultant. Then their manner changed. Of course, it shouldn't be that way, everyone should be treated with respect regardless of their seniority, but it was useful to be reminded of how hierarchies operate in the NHS. I resolved to make sure to support my junior colleagues when they were challenged.

Looking back now, I understand that this was an additional burden on me during what was already a very demanding time. And it made me doubt myself. I had to keep reminding myself of my capabilities. My impostor syndrome was hammering me – perhaps despite my years of working with infectious diseases, I just wasn't good enough for the role I found myself in? Impostor syndrome is often framed as the problem of the individual, and because of this, something the individual needs to resolve. Most weeks I receive emails from medical education companies, promising me that for a mere £150 plus VAT, I can attend an hour-long online course, to learn skills to increase my confidence and manage my impostor syndrome. But why do I feel like an impostor? And what if my impostor syndrome isn't 'all in my head', but rather something that has been fed back to me explicitly and implicitly throughout my life? What if the causes are structural? Should the solution then not be collective, rather than focused on the individual? I don't think we should have to pay to attend courses to get our impostor syndrome fixed.

Despite being a senior doctor with years of working in the NHS, I still felt like I wasn't being heard and taken seriously by my colleagues and members of the public. This is not unique to me – it is more likely to happen to women and people from minoritised groups and can have a huge impact on confidence and career progression. It can make us feel like we don't belong. Along with more overt forms of prejudice and discrimination, this contributes to more minoritised doctors leaving the healthcare workforce. This is not only harmful for the doctors involved, but for minoritised patients too, as a more diverse and inclusive workforce has been shown to improve patient care. To make healthcare services more welcoming for all patients, we need to make sure we do the same for doctors. We need to challenge the culture of exclusion that silences minoritised doctors to ensure that their patients are also heard.

*

It was after my mundane (and, I'm loathe to admit, still infuriating) Twitter incident, that I was introduced to testimonial injustice, which helped me to better understand my experience.[3] Testimonial injustice leads to patients not being heard, but it can affect minoritised doctors and anyone in the workplace too. Here's a common example of testimonial injustice at work, which you may recognise: you're in a meeting and you've just made what you think is a really astute point. You're basking in the glow of your own cleverness waiting for a response, maybe even praise, but nothing happens... tumbleweeds... the point is ignored by everyone. You're disappointed but get over it. The meeting moves on. A few minutes later, another more credible person makes the same point as you and gets the recognition you desired – you think to yourself, *See, it* was *a good point!* But because it was made by someone deemed to have more authority than you, it took their saying it for the point to be heard.

This has happened to me on countless occasions, will happen again, and is frustratingly predictable. Being a woman of colour puts me at increased risk of a credibility deficit, because of sexist and racist stereotypes widespread in society. It is important that I acknowledge here that I am middle class, cisgender, heterosexual and have no visible disabilities, which counteract this deficit. However, it's likely that repeated experiences of testimonial injustice, of not being heard, have contributed to my impostor syndrome. If I am not treated as a credible source of knowledge, is it any wonder that I feel like a fraud? Contrast this to white men, the group most likely to be seen as sources of authority when speaking – they are routinely given credence for knowing more than they might, something that is called a 'credibility excess'. You may be unsurprised to hear that white men are also the group least likely to report impostor syndrome.

When we are not listened to, it affects how we see ourselves – as humans capable of producing and passing on knowledge. If it happens repeatedly, we may lose some of our dignity and even some of our humanity. It can have a big impact on our self-esteem, and we may be less likely to speak up again in future meetings. Over our careers in the long-term, we may feel less confident to apply for promotions or leadership positions. In her book *The Authority Gap: Why Women Are Still Taken Less Seriously Than Men and What We Can Do About It*, Mary Ann Sieghart encapsulates some of the consequences of women being dismissed. She says, 'If women aren't taken as seriously as men, they are going to be paid less, promoted less and held back in their careers. They are going to feel less confident and less entitled to success.' She emphasises how inaction will mean that 'the gap between women and men in the public sphere will never disappear'.[4]

This causes a form of silencing that means that our unique points of view are unaired and lost from public discourse. As this happens more frequently to people from minoritised groups, this is particularly damaging – we lose a diversity of thought and leadership. This is bad for everyone, and in healthcare bad for patients. For doctors, this lack of confidence may mean not feeling capable enough to be on boards, such as those that decide policy and where funding should go. This has significant implications for health equity, as minoritised doctors are more likely to advocate for minoritised patients, and diseases that predominantly affect them. This can be seen when we look at the Black doctors and nurses who have transformed services for sickle cell disease. It's also no coincidence that I have a specialist clinical and research interest in the sexual health of British Asian women. When you are part of a group, you have a better understanding of its needs. You may recognise issues that people outside of the group wouldn't.

When minoritised doctors are excluded from leadership or decision-making boards, minoritised patient groups may not receive the funding or policy attention they need. This further reinforces historical patterns of marginalisation over the years.[5] An example of this is the health research gender gap in the UK, where despite a third of women experiencing a reproductive or gynaecological problem in their lifetime, less than 2.5 per cent of publicly funded research is allocated to this field.[6] This may be due to low representation of women on funding boards or fewer women holding senior positions over the years.

When doctors are unheard, the voices of their patients are less heard, exacerbating inequalities. The failure to listen to each other, and minoritised colleagues in particular, impacts *who* has the power to effect change in healthcare. Its roots lie deep in the core of what society deems a doctor 'should' look like, affecting their perceived authority.

*

A riddle:

> *A father and his son are in a car accident. The father dies. The son is rushed to the emergency department. The attending surgeon looks at the boy and says, 'I can't operate on this boy. He's my son!' How can this be?*

The surgeon is of course the boy's mother. This riddle originated on an American TV show and has been in common circulation for more than fifty years.[7] Did you get the right answer? If you did, you did better than 82 per cent of the 7,000 Americans asked in a study. Some of the more far-fetched answers included 'the boy was kidnapped by a man and raised to believe his kidnapper was his father' and 'the surgeon is a ghost'. Interestingly, women were no more likely to get the correct answer than men.

When you picture a doctor, what image comes to your mind? Perhaps it's someone who looks like you, your doctor, or maybe even someone who looks like me. But if you had searched 'doctor' on the internet just a few years ago, the most common image you would have found is of a white man. Medicine in Europe and America has long been white and male, reflecting inherent power structures in society. This is despite traditions in many different cultures around the world where women have been seen as the healers – administering remedies passed down through generations, responsible for nursing their families back to good health, delivering babies. With scientific advances in the nineteenth century, this traditional knowledge was swept aside. This transformation of medicine was seen as being male-orientated – the skills required to be a doctor being the 'male attributes' of technical competence and the ability to be objective. Male doctors deemed women lacking in these, due to their inherent nature and biology – such as being swayed by their hormones. We can see that the 'objective' assessments made at this time by male doctors were actually subjective and based on sexist attitudes rife in society.

It was not until the latter half of the twentieth century that numbers of female doctors started to catch up. This has been the case in many countries in the last few decades, particularly due to changes in societal gender norms. In the UK, since the formation of the NHS in 1948, recruitment of overseas doctors and nurses has been actively pursued to fill staffing gaps, leading to more people of colour in the workforce. However, the internet search and the surgeon riddle demonstrate just how deeply the stereotype of a white male doctor is embedded in society – in the case of the riddle, for many people imagining that a surgeon can be a woman is more ridiculous than the answers proffered.

In the UK, it was not until 1865 that Elizabeth Garrett Anderson became the first woman to qualify as a doctor and this was only by taking advantage of a loophole in the Worshipful Society of Apothecaries' admissions process.[8] However, she was unable to take up a post in any medical practice and had to set up her own. Immediately after realising their 'mistake', the Worshipful Society of Apothecaries* shamefully closed this loophole. It was only in 2021

---

*The Worshipful Society of Apothecaries of London is one of the livery companies (trade associations) of the City of London. It was founded in 1617 by apothecaries who were granted a Royal Charter. In 1815 it was given the power to license and regulate medical practitioners in England and Wales. Agatha Christie famously passed the Apothecaries Hall Assistants' Exam in 1917, to be a pharmaceutical assistant. No doubt this increased her knowledge of poisons, which would come in handy for future plot twists.

that the Worshipful Society appointed its second female Master, one of my mentors in HIV medicine, Professor Jane Anderson. The first was Professor Enid Taylor in 2002. The Worshipful Society now has a portrait of Dr Elizabeth Garrett Anderson hanging on their walls. In 1876, the Medical Act passed, which allowed for anyone regardless of gender to be licensed as a doctor, and in 1917 the Medical Women's Federation was founded. In the US, Elizabeth Blackwell was the first woman doctor, graduating in 1849. She went on to co-found the New York Infirmary for Women and Children.

Data from the Universities and Colleges Admissions Service (UCAS) show that now across the UK, more women than men start medical training. In 2016, 57 per cent of those accepted to medical school were women.[9] Despite this, women are under-represented in some medical specialities traditionally thought not to suit them, such as surgery where only one in eight consultants and a third of trainees are female.[10] Surgery has historically been seen as too physically tough for women to do (standing for hours, manipulating heavy limbs), with unsocial hours that don't fit in with caring for a family. There has also been the false perception that women don't have the right skills or the right personality to do surgery – they are too emotional to keep a cool head and steady hand under situations of extreme stress. This under-representation has led to several campaigns including one on social media where female surgeons have posted photos of themselves with the hashtag #ILookLikeASurgeon. This increased visibility broadens the public's imagination of who a surgeon can be and also means that aspiring female surgeons now have role models that look like them. The Royal College of Surgeons published a report into diversity in 2021 which highlighted the presence of an 'old boys' network' which was seen as a major barrier to leadership for those excluded from it.[11] More recently, surgery has been experiencing its own MeToo movement where female surgeons have felt empowered to speak up about their experiences of sexual harassment at work.[12] A recent report in the UK shockingly found that 30 per cent of women surgeons surveyed had been sexually assaulted by a co-worker.[13]

Despite efforts like #ILookLikeASurgeon, the idea that women aren't credible in these roles continues to be reinforced in popular culture and was highlighted during media coverage of the COVID-19 pandemic. Professor Claire Hopkins, a consultant ear, nose and throat (ENT) surgeon, took to Twitter to protest that during an interview on BBC News in 2021 she was introduced without her title, Professor. In contrast, the other interviewee, a male consultant ENT surgeon, Professor Nirmal Kumar, was given his title.[14] Incredibly this happened to her again in 2023.[15] On BBC's *Question Time* in June 2020, Professor Dame Donna Kinnair, the chief executive and general secretary of the Royal College of Nursing, had both her titles taken away, while Professor Hugh Pennington, bacteriologist at the University of Aberdeen, kept his. Professor Dame Kinnair is a Black British woman and Professor Pennington is a white British man.[16]

These are examples of what gender equity experts Amy Deihl and Leanne Dzubinski call 'untitling', a practice they say 'diminishes women's perceived authority and credibility'.[17] Not only are women more likely to be untitled, they are also less likely to untitle others. An American study showed that when female doctors introduce other female doctors when they are about to give a presentation, they used their titles almost every time. Male doctors only used female doctors' titles half of the time.[18] The authors said the reasons for this are unclear, but concluded that this was likely to amplify the 'isolation' and 'marginalisation' that female doctors experience. I think the reason is sexism. Women just aren't given the same amount of respect as their male colleagues for doing the same role. I can see how this can affect self-worth.

Women in medicine are marginalised and can face many difficulties in the workplace. A British Medical Association survey of its members in 2021 found that 84 per cent thought sexism was an issue in medicine. Of the female doctors responding, 91 per cent said they had experienced sexism at work, and 48 per cent said they felt they couldn't report it.[19] Sadly, women may also not feel safe at work. Surviving in Scrubs is a website set up by doctors where women can anonymously submit stories of sexism, sexual harassment and assault they have experienced in any NHS setting.[20] Similar to many professions, women also face a significant gender pay gap despite doing the same work as men. In England, the gap for hospital doctors is 11.9 per cent and GPs 15.3 per cent.[21] This shows again the lack of value afforded to women in the medical profession.

When white male doctors are viewed as 'the norm', what happens to everyone else? In the medical profession, I believe there is a culture of silencing and exclusion of people who don't fit traditional ideas of 'the norm' and this can affect their patients directly and indirectly.

*

Dr Sizer turned the ID card hanging on her lanyard so it was facing outwards again. It declared to the world that she, Dr Emma Sizer, was a consultant oncologist, a senior doctor who had completed specialist training and was an expert in cancer care. Even after three years, she still sometimes didn't quite believe this was her role, despite the almost twenty years of hard graft and clinical experience taken to get there.

'Moving on, quickly now! Who's next on the agenda?' Professor Eaves, clinical lead for urology, was chairing the cancer multi-disciplinary team meeting with his usual efficient steer.

These meetings aimed to discuss and plan the treatment of all patients in the local region with cancers affecting the kidneys, bladder, prostate gland and testicles. This week was particularly busy; they were trying to catch up with the backlog of cases after the COVID-19 pandemic, and still had ten patients to discuss in the next hour.

'It's Keith Asher,' answered the department administrator, skimming through the list in front of her.

'Thanks. Who's presenting him?' Professor Eaves asked the room.

'He's one of mine.' Dr Sizer took a deep breath and presented her patient's medical history.

Mr Asher was a 66-year-old man originally from Trinidad, who had emigrated to London in the 1970s, working as a bus driver for most of his adult life until he retired recently. He'd noticed some problems with passing urine for the last year, getting up five or six times a night and finding it difficult to fully empty his bladder. Although this meant he often had broken sleep, he'd ignored it, passing it off as something related to getting older. Since he'd retired, it was harder to dismiss and his wife had also noticed that he had started losing weight. Despite her best efforts to feed him up, cooking his favourite curry duck and roti, he'd lost 10kg. By now, he didn't need much persuading to agree to see his GP. Recognising that his symptoms sounded sinister, his doctor referred him onto the rapid access cancer pathway. Within weeks he'd had several investigations and been diagnosed with advanced prostate cancer, which had spread to his bones and liver. He was shocked when Dr Sizer broke the news to him in her clinic last week, holding onto his wife's hand tightly.

Dr Sizer finished presenting his case with her request. 'Mr Asher is aware his cancer is very advanced, and he realises he will die from it soon. He's getting his affairs in order. But his granddaughter is getting married in two months, and he is desperate to see her get wed. I've brought his case to this meeting to see if he may be eligible for that new therapy that's just been licensed. He's aware it won't cure him of the cancer, but it will slow it down so he gets a few extra months of quality time with his family and can go to the wedding.'

Dr Sizer exhaled and waited hopefully for a positive response from her colleagues. While she was used to working with cancer patients in her role as an oncologist, there was something about Mr Asher's case that had touched her deeply – maybe it was because he was a bus driver just like her dad. He too worked hard on low wages all his life, saving carefully for his retirement. He was now enjoying the rewards of this economy, spending the winter months in a timeshare apartment in sunny Alicante. In contrast, what did Mr Asher have left to look forward to, except for this family wedding before he died?

The cancer specialist nurse started off the discussion. 'Such a shame. To be diagnosed when the cancer is so far gone. And just when he should be allowed to relax and enjoy his retirement. I agree this is something we should seriously consider.'

The palliative care consultant concurred. 'Yes, really sad. Thanks for bringing him to the meeting. I'll take a note of his name and contact him to make sure his symptoms are under control. He's probably getting quite a bit of pain in his bones now. I agree, we should consider this new therapy. It will improve the quality of his last few months.'

Several other members of the multidisciplinary team nodded their heads in agreement.

Professor Eaves intervened. 'Yes, yes, this is a truly tragic case. But... we hear many of these sad cases. For whatever reason, he has waited until the cancer was very advanced before he sought help. I'm not sure this is the best option for him. Don't forget, the results of the trial showed the therapy was only partially effective in a minority of people. It didn't work so well in people at such an advanced stage of prostate cancer. And I hate to say it, but it is something we have to consider – it is very expensive and we are restricted in the number of people we can give it to.'

'You make some important points. Will it really help him at this late stage? And what about our other patients who may benefit more from it?' another consultant said.

The discussion continued for several minutes, reaching no definitive conclusion. Dr Sizer argued the case for her patient several times, trying to make sure she sounded measured, disguising the emotion in her voice. She felt the wave of opinion was turning away from her and her patient.

Professor Eaves cleared his throat. 'I know this is difficult, but we do need to reach a decision. We still have a lot of patients to discuss. In my opinion, we would be using a very expensive treatment on a patient in which there would be no clear benefit. We should save it for another patient whose cancer is less advanced and is in a better physical state. I think it's a "no", sorry to say. What do you all think?'

There was a pause. Then several nods.

'Dr Sizer?' He looked at her.

She thought about whether there was anything else she could say to sway them, but she had exhausted her options.

'Yes, OK,' she said quietly.

'OK, let's move on. Next patient?'

Dr Sizer sat in her seat feeling defeated. She was certain that just a few weeks ago, they had approved that same therapy for another patient – one who was frailer and whose cancer was more widespread.

He had been one of Robert's patients and Robert seemed to get whatever therapy he asked for at these meetings. He'd only been a consultant for a year, in comparison to her three, but came across much more confidently than she did. She once asked him about the secret of his success in these meetings and he said it was down to being a member of his debating club at school. And she thought cynically, his Oxbridge education, which he always managed to get into conversations. Professor Eaves had been at the same college as him, something they loved to chat about. People rarely disagreed with the professor, the most senior doctor in the department. If you could convince him of your case, you were more likely to get what you wanted for your patient.

Dr Sizer was the first person in her family to go to university, taking a substantial student loan and working various jobs to pay for her studies, while her peers were in the student bar. She was proud of where her conscientiousness had got her, but still found it galling to see how easily medical school had come to her friends. Many of them came from families full of doctors, and seemed to naturally understand the unspoken rules of NHS culture. Even now, she didn't have their self-assurance, often feeling like an outsider at work.

She thought to herself, *Could I have done more for Mr Asher? I'm so shy, and people, particularly the senior consultants, often talk over me. These meetings really are like attending a debate club. No wonder Robert is so good at it. People who talk more forcefully tend to get the treatment they want for their patients. Could I have been more assertive? I did remind them about that previous case, where the patient who was more unwell got the therapy, but when I mentioned it, no one said anything. It was like they ignored me. I'm not looking forward to giving Mr Asher more bad news . . .*

Multidisciplinary meetings like this one are held in many medical specialities. They are designed to make sure that the views of all of the professionals involved in a patient's care are considered. This is done with the acknowledgement that each staff member from a different discipline brings a different perspective, and this helps give a more holistic view of the patient. However, they only work when each member is heard. Patients can be directly affected when not *all* views are listened to or respected equally in meetings about their care.

I've had many experiences of multidisciplinary meetings during my career and seen how effective they can be when all views are considered. This describes the majority that I've attended, but I have also been to meetings where this doesn't happen. I've also had to learn how to be more assertive. I'm often asked to join meetings held by other specialist teams, as a patient's HIV doctor. The meeting is to discuss their suitability for treatment for a medical condition that may or may not be related to HIV. I bring my expertise in HIV medicine and my knowledge of the patient to the meeting. Importantly, I also advocate for the patient, as other doctors may not be up to date with HIV treatment advances and improvement in life expectancy. Astoundingly, patients living with HIV still face stigma and judgement from healthcare professionals, so I challenge this, should it come up. This is when it's particularly crucial that I speak up – a patient may not be deemed suitable for a therapy unless my view is heard. Over the years I have developed strategies to overcome my shyness and ensure this happens. I make sure I am fully prepared and up to date on the patient's condition and sometimes take a colleague with me for moral support. I find it helps to bring in the social context of a patient, essentially what makes them who they are, as it reminds everyone that the patient is more than their disease. I'm much more confident that I will be heard in meetings now, but this has meant going out of my comfort zone, practice and reflection.

In this scenario, Dr Sizer felt like she hadn't given a good enough case to support the new therapy for her patient. Unlike her more confident colleague, Robert, she found it difficult to be heard, despite her best efforts. Her working-class background sometimes made her feel like she didn't belong in the culture of the NHS which, like many workforces, has unspoken rules of behaviour. For example, she'd felt the need to refine her accent to sound like her privately educated colleagues. This, combined with a natural introversion, meant that she found it hard to speak up in lively discussions.

This feeling of not belonging has been described by sociologist Nirmal Puwar in her book *Space Invaders*.[22] She uses case studies to describe how professional spaces have been historically inhabited by bodies that are male and white, calling them 'the somatic norm'. Anyone who doesn't fit this bodily norm is seen to invade this space, hyper-visible to those who naturally occupy it. She terms them 'space invaders'. Space invaders have their capability continually doubted and they are often infantilised, treated as more junior than they are. They may feel that they are hired to fill a 'diversity' quota and bear a burden of representation. They are held up to higher standards of behaviour, pressurising them to work harder to be accepted. Space invaders are deemed not credible enough to belong to the workspace, creating a need to fit in, to mould themselves into somebody more acceptable. Puwar describes this as putting on a suit – one that is 'ill-fitting and unbecoming'. The daily effort of striving to fit in and to work harder to become an insider can be wearing and contribute to burnout. The notion of space invaders is clearly demonstrated in 'Broken Ladders', a joint report by the Fawcett Society and the Runnymede Trust which looked at the experiences of racially minoritised women across a range of employment sectors.[23] This found that in order to fit into the work environment, 61 per cent reported having to change themselves – their language, their hairstyle and even their name. This suggests that the change has to be made by those who don't fit in, rather than the culture that excludes them.

When doctors are not heard by their peers, this can have ramifications for patients. It can also affect their sense of belonging. They need to know that their voices are heard and valued equally, regardless of their background. They need to feel that their employer and colleagues care about them. Should Dr Sizer have to shout louder to be heard in these meetings, or should there be more effort made to make sure everyone is actively listened to and their views equally valued? Ideally, I believe that it should be about better listening, a skill that should be modelled by people in leadership positions.

Effective listening by leaders has been shown to make employees happier, more committed and less likely to leave.[24] Organisations become more efficient and creative. But what do employees regard as effective listening? Research shows that employees are more likely to report that they feel heard if they sense an openness during conversation with their managers, and if this leads to action. They feel unheard if their manager shuts them down, listens superficially and appears distracted.[25] Leaders also chair meetings where, as we've seen, incidents of testimonial injustice are common. To reduce this, meetings can be chaired in ways that intentionally ensure that everyone has a chance to speak, not just the loudest voices. I try to do this by letting everyone have a turn and even seeking the views of those more likely to be silent before the meeting. This makes sure all opinions are aired.

To me, this all comes down to making sure that people feel listened to and that their views and consequently their *selves* matter to an organisation. Leaders can also set an example in all areas of their work, by calling out negative behaviours, showing a willingness to be open to new perspectives and supporting minoritised members of the team through mentoring and coaching. Encouragingly, many leadership courses in the NHS now include training on how to practice inclusive behaviours, so that colleagues feel more heard. Every staff member can help their colleagues feel like they belong. However, leaders have a responsibility to do so. By modelling inclusive behaviours, they can set the culture of their workplace.

Beyond better listening, an important part of challenging what doctors should look like is role-modelling leaders from all backgrounds. I have been lucky to have such a role model. Professor Mala Rao is a public health doctor and academic based at Imperial College London, whose work in the UK and abroad has reduced health inequalities for countless people. She has held several international and national leadership positions and been at the forefront of culture change in the NHS. Rao was born in India and studied medicine in

Delhi. She moved to the UK to complete her post-graduate training in public health and became director of public health in Essex in the late 1980s. While there she investigated higher infant mortality rates in army families, which led to the provision of maternal social support. In other roles she established England's first evidence-based cancer network and led several public health workforce development innovations aimed at making public health everybody's responsibility.

More recently she has been focusing on the welfare of international medical graduates (IMGs). She has led on a new standardised induction to ensure they are welcomed, included and valued in the profession from the start. Rao is passionate about the knowledge that international medical graduates can bring from their work abroad, telling me that it is urgent that we learn from them. Many have experience of working in low- and middle-income countries and are experienced in delivering healthcare in resource-limited circumstances, which may be of increasing significance in a constrained NHS. However, she acknowledges that to date, 'the disappointing reality is that IMGs are seldom recognised for their potential to contribute to innovation and change, despite the fact that many will have ideas worthy of replication in an NHS setting'.

Like me, Rao is a woman of Indian heritage, and not only this, an international medical graduate. I asked her about her experiences of feeling excluded. She told me that she has had to develop strategies to be heard and taken seriously. This has included not being 'a victim of the erasure which so many of us experience, with our contributions remaining unacknowledged or worse still, being appropriated by others'. This has been 'against a background of bullying, intimidation and overt racism and discrimination which I have endured over a significant part of my career'.

Rao ensured she was so good at her job that there was no danger of criticism. She had been denied opportunities to have a career in academia so instead studied for a PhD in her own time while working as a full-time director of public health. In this way she felt she was directly challenging her bullies. The research studies that she has continued to carry out throughout her career are relevant to policy and have national impact, directly improving public health.

Rao said it was important for her to publish her findings and ensure her 'commitment and contributions to advance public health were not erased'. Rao also highlighted her collaborative and inclusive approach, identifying 'allies across professional and organisational boundaries, who may be better inclined to listen to my views'. She also told me about building 'a highly supportive network of friends and allies whose interventions have ensured that my views have been heard'. She emphasises that these include people of all genders and ethnicities.

As well as being a role model, Rao is one of my heroes. I feel some connection to her due to us both being medical women with roots in India and Essex. My mother even remembers seeing her speak at an evening lecture for GPs in the 1980s. Reflecting on my conversation with Rao, I think of the slogan 'If you can't see it, you can't be it.' She makes me feel hopeful that, like her, I can continue to speak up, highlight injustice and enact change to improve the health of marginalised communities.

*

In recent years, there has been increasing recognition that a culture of exclusion exists in healthcare systems. Consequently, there has been a drive to increase diversity in the workforce. In the NHS, there are many programmes aiming to promote the recruitment and retention of people from minoritised groups. There are good reasons for this. Firstly, the moral argument – all staff should be able to work in a culture where they feel safe and supported regardless of their background and social identities. Additionally, diverse organisations are more innovative, more productive, better at problem-solving and more efficient. Employees report greater engagement at work and are more likely to stay in their jobs. This is good for the sustainability of organisations in the long-term.[26]

Diversity can start at medical school. In their book *The Class Ceiling: Why it Pays to Be Privileged*, authors Sam Friedman and Daniel Laurison investigate how class affects who gets the most prestigious jobs in Britain. They found that medicine is one of the most elite professions with the highest over-representation of people from privileged backgrounds. It was also more likely to continually recruit people from the same backgrounds, limiting the diversity of doctors coming through the pipeline.[27] We've seen this in the scenario with Dr Sizer. Intervening at this stage is important. 'Widening participation' schemes focus on attracting and supporting a broader cohort of future doctors in their applications to medical school. These include, for example, students from racially minoritised backgrounds, those from deprived areas and those with a disability. This is done through workshops, mentoring and specific recruitment policies. Progress is also being made with the NHS bursary scheme, which means that students struggling with the cost of attending medical school are better supported financially.[28]

Dr Enam Haque, a GP and specialist in widening participation at the University of Manchester Medical School, helped to set up the National Medical Schools Widening Participation Forum in 2015, a collaborative organisation of medical schools, voluntary organisations, medical students and junior doctors. It aims to increase the proportion of students from underprivileged backgrounds who gain entry to a medical school and successfully complete the course. He told me that he was passionate about this because he himself was from such a background, growing up in a poor mining town in Yorkshire. His father owned a restaurant and worked hard to pay for him to go to medical school. Once he got there, he noticed the 'huge disparities between those from wealthy and those from less wealthy backgrounds' and 'felt an outsider during my studies'. He complained to the director of admissions about the low levels of diversity and was given the first-ever widening participation lead role in the medical school. I asked him about what effect the National Medical Schools Widening Participation Forum has had so far. He replied, 'It provides a voice for those who want to address the inequalities in medical education.' I later found out that my hospital was running an initiative to assist underprivileged A-level students in the area to access work experience placements. This is essential for medical school applications but is difficult to arrange unless you know somebody who works in the NHS. In fact, that's how I got my work experience placement – through my GP mother.

NHS organisations that have fewer minoritised staff reporting negative workplace experiences tend to have higher patient satisfaction.[29] Seeing a doctor who looks like you may make them seem more approachable. They may share a similar cultural background to you and so be better able to understand who you are and where you are coming from. You may feel more comfortable with them, more able to ask questions, more likely to believe what they say and to take their advice. There is increasing evidence to show a diverse workforce is better for the health of patients.

A study by researchers in California investigated whether Black men would be more likely to take up health prevention services if they had Black male doctors.[30] Black men were recruited from barbershops and flea markets in Oakland for a health consultation and assigned to either a Black male doctor or a non-Black male doctor. Those that had a Black doctor were more likely to agree to get their blood pressure measured, to have a blood test for diabetes, or a flu vaccine – all important measures to prevent serious disease. There was also an improvement in mistrust. Black men who expressed mistrust with healthcare services at the start of the study, were more likely to change their mind about health prevention services if they talked to a Black doctor. The study team predicted that if there were more Black doctors in the workforce, there would be an incredible 8 per cent reduction in the gap in life expectancy between Black and white men in the US.

This was reinforced by another US study published in 2023 that showed that in counties with more Black primary care physicians, Black residents had a longer life expectancy and lower mortality.[31] These are stark results backed up by more research. Several studies have shown that matching the gender and ethnicity of the patient and the doctor improved rates of cancer screening and increased the number of patients seeking and using healthcare services.[32, 33] Having a Black doctor in pregnancy has been found to lead to better health outcomes for newborn Black babies.[34]

However, not all studies show that matching a doctor's ethnicity or gender to a patient's improves their experience. This may be more commonly seen in stigmatised health conditions. In sexual health, for example, patients from minoritised groups may prefer to see someone from outside their community, due to concerns about confidentiality. It's likely that patients value more than just whether their doctor looks like them. A study found that patients who felt they shared similar personal beliefs, values and ways of communicating with their doctors thought they had a stronger relationship. They were more likely to trust them, to feel satisfied with their care, and to take their medication.[35] This is particularly important when you consider that half of patients with chronic illnesses do not take their medication as prescribed.[36]

For patient care, increasing the diversity of staff may improve health outcomes. However, it's not a panacea – the NHS is already one of the most diverse organisations in the UK and yet minoritised patients and staff still report discrimination. It seems vital to make sure that *all* staff are trained to provide care to patients that is without prejudice or discrimination. Representation cannot resolve everything; all should be able to listen to and care for all patients with dignity and respect. For patients, critically this means that they will have doctors who are better able to *hear* them, to *understand* their needs and to *advocate* for them.

*

I'd taken ages getting ready that morning. My black leather shoes were shiny with polish, my thick, usually unruly hair had been smoothed into a high ponytail, my new trousers and shirt were freshly pressed. I was seventeen years old and it was my first day of work experience in the NHS. This was the day I hoped would be a step towards a lifetime's work as an NHS doctor. I'd been told by school careers advisors that getting work experience would be essential in my application for a place on a medical degree course. Knowing this was highly competitive, it seemed like a sensible thing to do. I was to shadow Dr Hillier, a consultant in the emergency department of my local hospital for two days. I was excited and nervous.

I spent the morning accompanying Dr Hillier as he assessed, reviewed and treated patients attending the department. I was incredibly impressed by his skills: he seemed able to take in multiple sources of information before coming up with a provisional diagnosis and management plan. By the afternoon, I was exhilarated and a little overwhelmed – was this a job that I would ever be capable of doing? Dr Hillier seemed to hold a wealth of medical knowledge, and not only that, with his years of experience, he appeared to always know exactly the right thing to do at the right time. He maintained an aura of calm, despite the frenetic environment of the emergency department. In contrast, the managed chaos in the department raised my adrenaline levels, causing my heart to beat slightly faster all day. The patients had started to blur into one.

Dr Hillier was carrying out a long post-lunch round of the patients who were awaiting a decision on whether they were to be admitted or discharged. Together with the charge nurse, we stopped outside cubicle 10. Dr Stevens, the registrar, looked at his notes and started to present the patient waiting for us inside.

'This is Mr Smith, a 67-year-old smoker with a history of emphysema. He complains of five days of worsening shortness of breath, initially on exertion and now at rest. This is associated with a cough productive of yellow sputum and mild fever. He has no night sweats, chest pain or ankle swelling. He has been using his inhalers regularly, but they no longer help. Observations are stable on 2 litres of oxygen. ECG is normal. My impression is that he has a chest infection, which has worsened his emphysema. I am waiting on blood results and a chest x-ray to look for pneumonia. Apart from oxygen, I have given him some antibiotics, steroids and nebulisers. I think he will need to stay in for a couple of days and have already referred him to the admitting medical team.'

Dr Hillier voiced his assent. 'Excellent work. That sounds like a sensible plan. Shall we go in?'

Not waiting for an answer, he swept aside the curtains dividing the cubicle from the next and strode in. We followed him into the cubicle, and arranged ourselves around the patient, who was lying on a hospital trolley.

Mr Smith was a slight man, his skin pale and sweaty. Propped up by several pillows, he was taking shallow breaths from an oxygen mask covering his face. His cheeks looked flushed and his eyes were bulging as he warily looked up at us standing around the bed.

'Hello, Mr Smith, is it? I'm Dr Hillier, one of the consultants working in this department. Dr Stevens has just been telling us what's brought you in here. How are you feeling now?'

There was silence.

Leaning down towards the patient, in a louder voice, Dr Hillier repeated the question, 'How are you feeling, Mr Smith?'

A pause. Then the patient glared at him and suddenly bawled, 'Sorry, I can't have this. I'm OK with you all here . . . but not her . . . she needs to leave. She's making me feel worse!'

It was only when he lifted his finger to point, did I realise it was me he was talking about. The rest of the team followed his finger, turning their gaze towards me.

'It's just not on. I'm not having a P*** in here. She needs to get out. You, yes you, you need to get out!' By the end of his racist rant, he was shouting.

I couldn't believe this was happening to me. My feet were stuck to the ground, but I felt as if I was watching the scene from afar. This was something that happened in TV dramas, or to other people. *It couldn't be happening to me.* I waited to see what was going to happen next. Surely, the patient would be reprimanded for using such a heinous racist slur on me?

Dr Hillier looked panicked, then said softly to me, 'Perhaps it would be better if you leave. We'll catch up later.'

As I made to leave, the charge nurse whispered, 'Go to the staff room and have a cup of tea and a biscuit. Some time out. I'll come and find you later.' She smiled kindly and turned back to the patient.

Humiliated, I fled the cubicle, eventually finding my way to the staff room. I had only been called that slur once before in my seventeen years. It was yelled at me by a younger child while I was walking home from school. I had dismissed it at the time, believing the boy didn't really know what it meant. This, however, was clearly intended, and it shook me to my core – was this what it was going to be like working in the NHS? What was I letting myself in for?

To date, the NHS had always provided me with a sense of home; I felt like I grew up in it. Both of my parents had worked in the NHS all their lives – my mother as a GP and my father as a dentist. Their hours were long, with frequent weekend and evening clinics. They carefully juggled work with childcare and school pickups. At least once a week, my sister and I spent an evening in one of their surgeries, doing our homework or reading until they finished work. Once, one of my father's regular patients noticed I was studying with my books spread on the floor of the staff room, so he built me a desk that I could use when I was there. I am still touched by this significant act of unprompted kindness.

This experience of being racially abused on my first day of work experience made me question my relationship with the NHS. It no longer felt so welcoming. I had got my work experience placement easily due to my privilege of being from a medical family, but the episode of racism I describe shows how although I was advantaged in some ways, I wasn't in others. It didn't put me off applying to medical school, and I have never been called a racist slur at work again. Curiously, I had forgotten about this incident until I started writing this book. I'm not sure why. Perhaps as it was such a formative experience, it was too traumatic to remember; perhaps at the time I felt this was just another work difficulty that NHS staff had to put up with; perhaps it was because I never experienced such overt racism again. In any case, looking back I feel desperately sad for seventeen-year-old me, so excited to start her career. I feel anger at how the medical team acquiesced to the patient's wishes and, to my knowledge, did not later challenge him. I would now expect the medical team to behave differently, as racial abuse targeted at staff is no longer tolerated in the NHS. The patient would be told that such language was unacceptable and be given at least a verbal warning. However, in the late 1990s it was allowed.

When I talked to my parents about their experiences of racism in the NHS, they had much to say. My parents were part of a wave of healthcare professionals that were called from the former British colonies in Asia, the Caribbean and Africa to staff the newly formed NHS after the Second World War. An estimated 18,000 doctors came from the Indian subcontinent between the 1940s and 1980s and many ended up working in deprived areas and in unpopular specialties such as general practice, psychiatry and geriatrics. Many have reported experiencing racism.[37] Currently a quarter of NHS staff are from racially minoritised backgrounds, and due to vacancies, recruitment is still needed from overseas.[38] This has been called a 'brain drain' – a rich country divesting poorer countries of their medical workforce.

My parents recall incidents in the seventies of being told by patients that they wanted to see a 'proper' doctor/dentist, not them. And it wasn't only patients. An anaesthetist told my mother in her first house officer job that unless she left the operating theatre, he would not proceed with anaesthetising the patient. She had no choice but to leave.

However, my parents also talk fondly about the British colleagues who went out of their way to support them. For my mother, the consultant who taught her how to carry out colposcopy procedures and for my father, the senior dentist who provided him with references from his first clinical attachment so that he could apply for jobs. The NHS also offered us extended family. We had few relatives in the UK, and so my 'aunties' and 'uncles' were my parents' friends from work, medical and dental school, who'd also migrated. We'd meet them at weekends, at their houses or ours – an opportunity to share the languages, food and music of the homes we'd left behind.

While I've given examples of racism from several decades ago, racial prejudice and other forms of discrimination are still experienced by healthcare staff from colleagues and patients. This makes me sad and angry. It ranges from overt slurs to more subtle acts of exclusion. It continues to exert a considerable emotional toll. The British Medical Association, the largest doctors' union in the UK, surveyed its members in 2021. They reported that more than three quarters had experienced racism in the workplace in the last two years. This was most common for doctors who had trained overseas. Six in ten (60 per cent) of those experiencing racism said it had negatively affected their mental health and self-confidence, leaving them feeling frustrated, demotivated and angry. Many were considering leaving or had left their jobs because of it.[39] It's not only doctors. A survey published by the Royal College of Nursing in the UK in 2021 reported that racism was rife in the nursing workforce. White nurses were twice as likely to get promoted as Black and Asian staff. Black nurses working in hospitals and in the community were more likely to report having experienced physical abuse from patients than nurses from other ethnic backgrounds.[40]

In an effort to address racism, in 2015 the NHS Workforce Race Equality Standard, a compulsory reporting system for all hospitals in England, was implemented. It aims to 'close the gap in workplace experience between white and Black, Asian and minority ethnic colleagues'.[41] It has found that racially minoritised doctors are under-represented at consultant level and in academic posts. They are more likely than white staff to report harassment, bullying, abuse and discrimination from colleagues. They are also twice as likely to be disciplined and referred to the General Medical Council, where they may have their license to practice reviewed. This is truer for international medical graduates. White staff members are more likely to be appointed if short-listed for a promotion, have more training opportunities and believe they have more chances of career progression.

To understand how this discrimination operates among health-care staff, researchers from King's College London published a paper appropriately titled 'They created a team of almost entirely the people who work and are like them'.[42] They interviewed forty-eight healthcare workers in London, finding that racial hierarchies among staff were common, with white staff at the top holding the most power. This order was reinforced by prejudices and negative racial stereotypes leading to microaggressions, bullying, discrimination and harassment. Unsurprisingly, this negatively affected work perform-ance, staff experience and their health. Such experiences can also be seen in other countries in the West, for example in the US where Black female workers are over-represented in the healthcare sector, but usually in poorly paid caring roles.[43] There is also a significant ethnicity pay gap, with Black doctors being paid less than their white counterparts.[44]

Other forms of discrimination are also experienced by healthcare staff in the NHS. This includes disabled doctors who report fear of being treated unfavourably if they disclose their disability, and have difficulties accessing working environments that have not been designed with them in mind.[45] A survey of LGBTQ+ doctors and medical students in 2016 found high levels of harassment, but also under-reporting of this.[46] People also face prejudice due to their religion. For example, female Muslim doctors have reported discrimination within dress code polices, such as not being allowed to wear head scarves in operating theatres.[47]

These experiences are not unique to healthcare settings. However, the NHS is the largest employer in the UK, employing 1.5 million people in England, or one in nineteen workers. As a result, it is sometimes referred to as 'a microcosm of society' and so inherently holds many of society's attitudes, including its prejudices. Like many workplaces, the NHS does not always provide a safe and nurturing culture for all of its employees. It is estimated that bullying and harassment costs the NHS a staggering £2 billion a year in sickness, legal costs and staff turnover.[48] Challenging bad behaviours would be cost-effective, as well as good for staff wellbeing and ultimately patients. I think it is ironic that a service that has been specifically created to provide care to people can be so uncaring to the people who work for it – and this needs to change.

*

In 2009, the NHS Constitution for England declared that the NHS must 'make sure nobody is excluded, discriminated against or left behind'.[49] Since then, there has been a drive to improve staff and patient experience in the NHS.

In recent years, NHS trusts have started to introduce courses for staff as part of their strategies to improve equality, diversity and inclusion. Among these are courses to improve cultural competency and reduce unconscious bias. However, there is little evidence to show that these have had an impact on reducing discrimination against colleagues and patients from minoritised backgrounds.[50] Courses to address impostor syndrome are also becoming more common. I spoke to Rita, an NHS employee who attended one as part of her management training. She said that while the course was 'an interesting space to reflect', the most useful thing for her was to 'see how many other people suffered from it'. This suggests that tackling impostor syndrome includes recognising its pervasiveness. Such courses should also acknowledge that it's not the fault of the person experiencing it, and that there is a need to work collectively to address it. A more useful course that I have attended is Active Bystander training, which teaches people how to respond when witnessing discrimination.[51] It gives clear actions on how to support the victim, and challenge unacceptable behaviour. This is a practical framework that encourages people to speak up and be allies.

Fundamentally I believe that we must recognise that it's not just about addressing the behaviour of a 'few bad apples'. There is a culture of silencing and exclusion that all healthcare workers contribute to. We all have a responsibility to change it, and leaders in particular. Additionally, while individuals create policies and contribute to workplace culture, courses aimed at changing individual behaviours are not enough, we need institutional and systemic change. The political activist, academic and writer Angela Davis spoke at the University of California in 2015 about this, saying that it's not enough just to make organisations more diverse. 'It's a difference that doesn't make a difference. Diversity without structural transformation simply brings those who were previously excluded into a system as racist, as misogynistic, as it was before.'[52]

*

There are many ways in which structural transformation can occur in the NHS and other healthcare systems. These include:

- Appointing senior leaders that are diverse and represent the communities their hospitals serve. This could be encouraged through affirmative action such as mentoring schemes for staff from minoritised backgrounds to encourage them to apply for leadership positions, and to support them when they get there.

- Ensuring procedures for recruitment and promotion are fair and transparent. Methods to reduce bias such as listing objective criteria when hiring for a position, and blind short-listing (so applicants' personal details are hidden) should be used.
- Implementing action plans to improve workplace experiences for minoritised staff. For example: strategies on tackling racism, homophobia and transphobia, policies on parental leave and the gender pay gap, improving accessibility for disabled staff.
- An anonymous process for staff to report incidents of bullying and discrimination, so they do not fear retribution. Support should be provided to people who have experienced prejudice from colleagues or patients. This should include evidence that action has been taken.
- Staff should also have safe spaces where they can talk freely to peers, without fear of being disciplined. Examples of this in my hospital include networks for women, ethnic minorities, LGBTQ+ staff, disabled staff, and these are popular with employees.
- Monitoring data on issues such as employee recruitment, pay and progression opportunities, employee perceptions of fairness and inclusion. This would pick up inequalities between groups and hopefully initiate action.
- Accountability and even sanctions for poorly performing organisations. For example, those that score badly on markers of staff experience such as racial bullying or poor career progression, should be held accountable and pushed to make changes. In England, health and social care organisations are regularly inspected by the Care Quality Commission and are rated on a scale between 'Outstanding' and 'Inadequate'. Data on discrimination is not currently included as part of the criteria for this rating. Perhaps if it were, staff experience would be made a higher priority by employers.

It's heartening to see change happen. For example, in the last few years we have seen healthcare leaders from minoritised backgrounds rise to top positions at NHS England, the British Medical Association and the NHS Race and Health Observatory. We're now seeing leaders who are more relatable to a greater breadth of the workforce, who also seem to want to create transformational change. This doesn't always happen – I have witnessed in several different areas of medicine, female and minoritised leaders who have pulled the ladder up after them or perpetuated bullying behaviours that exclude. I have also seen many inspiring leaders like Professor Mala Rao who have made positive changes happen, and they give me hope for the future. Conversations about inclusion are now much more common. People are recognising the impact of prejudice on minoritised staff and patients. These are encouraging signs that a shift in healthcare workplace culture is happening, but this momentum needs to continue at pace, be funded and be sustainable.

I've been inspired to get involved in this shift too. In 2022, I co-led an investigation into equity, equality, diversity and inclusion at the British HIV Association, and now chair the working group that is acting on its findings. We aim to make more members of the association, along with the HIV community it serves, feel included and integral to its work. I'm proud to be part of this and hope that we will achieve our ultimate goal – of improving the health of people living with HIV in the UK.

*

In the end, my Twitter thread on racial health disparities in the UK did have the effect I wanted. It sparked considerable conversation on medical Twitter about racism and health and I was asked to write an opinion piece for a medical journal, *BMJ Leader*.[53] In it, I made the case that for decades the health needs of racially minoritised communities in the UK have been disregarded and under-prioritised. I posed the question, 'Can a healthcare system in which the disparities listed above exist over decades be said to be valuing all human life equally?'

As one of my solutions, I suggested that 'listening and valuing the voices of those most disadvantaged in our society' is essential. This is an argument that I have continued to think about since and I realise has been a substantial part of my journey towards writing this book. I was also supported to develop my book proposal through a widening participation scheme for new non-fiction writers from the Wellcome Collection and Spread the Word organisations.

Patient care suffers when doctors don't listen to each other. Ensuring minoritised doctors and healthcare workers are heard and valued is important for the health of minoritised patients. A healthcare workforce that is diverse, where everyone feels included, leads to happier and more productive employees, who are more likely to stay in the organisation. This is cost-effective, as well as good for patients and organisations.

Summary: How minoritised doctors can be better heard

- For individuals:
  - Reflect on your own listening practice, biases and blind spots. Let yourself be curious and open to what people tell you. Foster humility – perhaps other people have valid things to say? Think about how well you listen to your colleagues – do you let them speak and do you take them seriously. If not, why not?
  - Learn how to be an active bystander and speak up when you see bullying or discrimination.
  - If you find it difficult to be heard, think about what you can do to improve this. This could include making sure you are prepared for meetings, dressing in a way that makes you feel more confident, taking a course in assertiveness.

- For healthcare leaders:
  - Model an inclusive culture that challenges bullying and discrimination.
  - Chair meetings in a way that means all voices are heard. Ask less forthcoming members of the group for their opinion before the meeting if needs be.
  - Encourage reflection and supervision in your team and show that you do this yourself.
  - Bring up people after you – mentor and coach, or provide opportunities for your staff to access this.

- For healthcare organisations and government:
  - Diversify leadership through mentoring schemes and transparent recruitment processes that are unbiased.
  - Put equity at the heart of policy including implementing action plans to improve workplace experiences for minoritised staff.

- o Tackle bullying and discrimination from staff and patients, and support workers who have experienced it.
- o Provide safe spaces for staff to feed back and to talk to peers.
- o Monitor data on employee recruitment, pay and progression opportunities, employee perceptions of fairness and inclusion. Take action if inequalities are found.
- o Ensure accountability and even sanctions for poorly performing organisations on equity, diversity and inclusion.

4

Missing

How Silencing Causes a Knowledge Gap

November 1998.

It must be lunchtime, Alan thinks. He can smell boiled carrots and peas, their aroma barely masking the pervasive stench of bleach and body fluids. It's making him feel slightly sick. He hopes the doctors will get to him on their round soon. The ward around him hums with activity, staff going through their daily machinations. He's been there for six weeks now and feels like he knows the routine well. How much his life has changed in that small period of time!

Six weeks ago, he'd been at work as normal, leading his weekly Monday morning team meeting. They'd been working on a campaign for an important client and the pressure was mounting. But he was optimistic that what they were producing was high quality – he just needed to keep his colleagues enthused for a bit longer to get the campaign over the finishing line. That morning he'd felt a little under the weather, but ignored it – he'd slept poorly and he needed to be 100 per cent at work. As he stood addressing his team, he thought about how much he loved this part of his job – four decades in advertising and the thrill of a big project still excited him.

That's the last thing he can remember. The next is lying on the floor of the office, looking up at the faces of his concerned colleagues. He later found out that he had suddenly stopped mid-flow and collapsed. An ambulance was called and he was sped, alarms blaring, blue lights flashing, to hospital. The next few hours were a blur, but he'll never forget the doctor telling him and his wife that the diagnosis was a stroke. Tests had shown that a blood clot had travelled up from his heart and blocked an artery in his brain, starving part of it of blood and oxygen. This meant he was unable to move the right side of his face and body, and when he tried to speak, he struggled to find words.

Since then, he had been on this ward having regular physical therapy and waiting to see how much function he could recover. He had been started on a daily handful of pills to try and prevent a second stroke – medicine to control his blood pressure, regulate his heartbeat, reduce his cholesterol and thin his blood. There'd been some improvement, but he was unable to walk without help and communication was still difficult. When he looked in the mirror, it was hard to recognise himself. He looked like he had aged a couple of decades and the right side of his face drooped, the muscles starting to slacken from under-use. And it was all so frustrating! He shouldn't be there. This was not what he had planned for this stage in his life.

The metallic clang of the medical notes trolley indicated that the doctors had arrived. They swept the curtains around his bed to give the illusion of privacy and surrounded him, imposing in their white coats. The most junior doctor balanced Alan's thick folder in his arms, fountain pen poised to document the discussion. The consultant, Dr Kapoor, gave him a broad smile, declaring, 'Good news! Funding has been approved for the rehabilitation hospital. We hope they will have a vacant bed in the next couple of weeks so you can be transferred there for ongoing therapy. Hopefully just a short stay there and you'll be home soon.'

Was this 'good news'? Alan thought. *Another hospital, a bit more therapy, but no one could tell him if he could walk again. If he'd be able to live independently again. He was only sixty-three! He didn't want to spend the rest of his life being a burden to his wife and kids. What did he have left to look forward to?*

He forced himself to listen to the doctors, but he could feel that he was sinking deeper into depression. His life had changed dramatically in just a few minutes. He had to accept this and move on for the sake of his family, but for now, he wanted to let himself wallow a little bit longer.

I cared for many patients like Alan when I was working in general medicine as a junior doctor. The focus then was on recovery and preventing another stroke, as there was little else that we could do. While both remain important today, the management of strokes has dramatically changed in the intervening years. Alan would have a very different experience now. In the last two decades, advances in the care of patients who have experienced a stroke have dramatically changed their prognosis. This has included improved knowledge of what happens to the body when having a stroke, better scans and early intervention with treatment. If the stroke is due to a blood clot, this can now be dissolved with medication if given within four hours of the patient developing symptoms. This requires members of the public to be able to recognise the symptoms of a stroke quickly and contact emergency services, so educational campaigns have been developed to help with this. In the UK, this is the FAST campaign with the letters standing for Face droops, Arm weakness, Speech difficulty and Time is critical. Stroke doctors now work on an on-call rota so they can assess patients at any time of day for this urgent treatment. Clots can also be removed using new surgical techniques. Patients are now more likely to be admitted to a stroke unit so they get the specialised care they need. Rehabilitation is now more intensive and starts earlier, as soon as the patient is stabilised, and can be continued at home if safe.

All of these interventions together mean that the long-term damage to the brains and bodies of stroke patients is greatly reduced. If Alan had his stroke in 2023, he would have hugely benefited from this knowledge, which exists due to the research done in the intervening twenty-five years. Stroke is an example of a knowledge gap which has been filled. This has been done because policymakers and researchers have prioritised it, realising funding and resources were needed to improve care. Strokes can affect anyone but are more common in people with high blood pressure, raised cholesterol, diabetes, who smoke and who have a family history of stroke. It's great to see so much progress, and I'm sure there will be more to come.

In contrast, research gaps in the conditions that predominantly affect minoritised groups in society take much longer to fill. This is due to the silencing of minoritised researchers at multiple stages of the research process. These researchers will often study conditions that affect people from their communities, so when they are not heard, these diseases are not prioritised, and the research is not done. This contributes to gaps in our collective medical knowledge and it is minoritised patients who suffer, from a lack of effective investigations, treatment and care. An example of this is sickle cell disease, a condition that mainly affects Black people and where until recently, there has been little progress in effective therapies. The silencing of minoritised researchers happens within research institutions, but also on a much wider global scale. This is linked to enduring beliefs that some people's lives have less value than others. I've been affected by a research gap in my own life.

*

For me, the condition was endometriosis. Once I was diagnosed, I couldn't believe that despite it being 2018, almost one hundred years since endometriosis was first named, experts were still deliberating whether it was one disease or several. I discovered this at the first UK scientific conference on endometriosis run for the public, by the charity Endometriosis UK, with the Wellcome Trust. While I was used to going to conferences in my professional life, this was my first as a patient. I was excited to learn about the latest research and eager for any advice that might help me face daily life with the condition. Most importantly, I wanted to be in a space where endometriosis was talked about, no longer a disease of silent and solitary suffering, but one shared by many. At the first session I sat in the lecture hall so packed with people, some were sitting on the floor in the aisles. I could feel the energy fizzing around the room. This felt like a significant moment – more than 200 people gathering on a Saturday in their free time, our collective aim to tackle this pernicious disease.

Endometriosis is a common gynaecological condition experienced by more than 176 million people around the world. This includes approximately 1 in 10 cisgender women, with the numbers of transgender men and non-binary people who menstruate unknown. In endometriosis, cells similar to those lining the womb (endometrial cells) are found elsewhere in the body, such as the pelvis, bowel and bladder. During the menstrual cycle, endometrial cells build up, thickening the lining of the womb to prepare it for a possible pregnancy. If this doesn't happen, the lining breaks down, causing bleeding which is seen as a period. With endometriosis, the cells outside of the womb act in the same way, but the blood is unable to leave the body, causing inflammation and scarring. This can cause painful periods, chronic pelvic pain, pain during or after sex, fatigue, painful bowel movements and urination. While endometriosis is not life-threatening, it is hugely debilitating, having profound and long-lasting impacts on people's health and quality of life. It is one of the most common causes of infertility. I was diagnosed with endometriosis at the age of thirty-one. My journey to diagnosis was an unusual one, but it illustrates how it has been under-prioritised in medicine for a very long time, as a condition that predominantly affects women.

It all began with our decision to have a baby. On an unusually glorious Sunday afternoon in late spring, we took the opportunity to go for a drink in our local pub garden. Cars were driving past blaring dance music from open windows; the sky was cloudless and that kind of blue where everything and anything felt possible. This included becoming parents. As we made a toast, grinning at each other in thrall of the momentous decision we had made, I can remember musing that my pint may be one of the last alcoholic drinks I'd be having for a while. The next day, I came off the contraceptive pill and in excitement we waited, expecting to get pregnant immediately.

But nothing happened.

Each month my period arrived. I noticed they were starting to get more and more painful. Worried, I went to my GP who arranged an ultrasound scan to check I didn't have a cyst in my ovaries. They found nothing abnormal and no plans for further tests were made. I was relieved, but not completely reassured that everything was OK. After all, I wasn't pregnant yet and I had started to dread the cramps and lower back pain that accompanied my monthly bleed. I decided to keep an eye on my symptoms and see how things progressed.

I confess my symptom monitoring was less rigorous than it could have been. Life took over – I had post-graduate exams to revise for and was planning a joint thirtieth birthday celebration with a friend. But I couldn't ignore my body's shouts to be heard any longer. One evening after visiting a potential birthday venue, I was in so much pain I could barely walk home from the station. This was despite having taken two different types of painkiller, which I had gotten used to taking daily. As I gingerly shuffled home, I realised *this wasn't normal.* I resolved to make another appointment with the doctor. But before I could do this, it felt like the universe intervened and my diagnosis became clear to me.

As part of my specialist training in sexual health medicine, I was required to observe gynaecology clinics. That afternoon it was a clinic for women with chronic pelvic pain. The consultant was an experienced gynaecologist with a reassuring manner. I settled into my seat, my mind on my weekend plans. I was woken from my inertia by the first patient, a young woman in her early thirties. She seemed to be telling *my* story. Astonished, I listened to her narrate how her periods had become intensely painful after coming off the pill to get pregnant, and how this still hadn't happened after months of trying. I leant forward, as eager as the patient to hear the consultant's verdict.

'I think you may have endometriosis,' he suggested.

He went on to explain that as the oral contraceptive pill is a treat-ment for endometriosis, being on it can often mask its symptoms. When people come off the pill, they can develop painful periods. As he arranged investigations for her, I sat through the rest of the clinic stunned. Recurrent thoughts kept looping around my mind: *Did I have endometriosis? And if so, why hadn't I thought of it earlier?* I realised it was a condition I knew very little about as our teach-ing on it was minimal at medical school. However, I couldn't help berating myself for not suspecting it sooner and enduring what was, by now, more than a year of pain and dashed hopes of conceiving.

At my appointment with the family doctor, I was able to name endometriosis as my main concern, and they referred me to gynae-cology there and then. Three months later I had keyhole surgery which confirmed that I had Stage 4 disease, the most serious kind. This had wreaked havoc to my insides, sticking my bowel to my uterus, twisting my fallopian tubes until they were impassable. As I came round from the anaesthetic, the surgeon gently told me I was unlikely to get pregnant naturally and referred me to the fertility clinic, where our in vitro fertilisation (IVF) journey began.

Several years, four cycles of IVF, three further operations, two fallopian tubes removed and a traumatising hospital admission with pain later, we decided to stop trying to conceive. It was too physically and mentally distressing. My body was rejecting the daily injections, I was bloated and in pain, my mind rejecting the cycles of hope and desolation. I started hormonal treatment to control my symptoms and stop my periods until I reached menopause. This wasn't straightforward and it took me a while to find a combina-tion that suited me. First I tried monthly injections that threw me precipitously into menopause and though I found the sudden hot flushes and mood swings just about bearable, the forgetfulness made me worry I couldn't function on a day-to-day level. I had to write everything down, to make sure it wasn't missed. Eventually I was able to find a combination of hormones and lifestyle advice with side effects I could tolerate.

Now, my endo lives with me, an unwelcome guest in my unwill-ing body. I picture it as a small demonic Pac-Man, mostly asleep, but occasionally waking to remind me it still exists. On those days when I am exhausted and in pain, a hot water bottle and ibuprofen are my best friends. Infertility has been harder to come to terms with, a journey I am still taking, but I have come to realise that mothering can come in many different forms.[1]

I count myself lucky – my diagnosis only took two years. The average time to an endometriosis diagnosis in the UK is eight years, a wait so long I feel furious just writing it.[2] I went to my GP and my concerns were taken seriously; my doctor privilege meant that my symptoms were believed. I knew what language I needed to use to get the tests and referrals I needed. In a way, I was the 'ideal patient' that I discuss in Chapter 2, describing a medical history that 'fit' the possible diagnosis of endometriosis. But why did it take a chance hearing about endometriosis for me to think about it? Why didn't my GP or I suspect endometriosis sooner, before it become so advanced?

I suspect one of the reasons is that endometriosis and other gynaecological conditions have historically received little space on the medical school curriculum. Teaching on 'women's health' generally covered just pregnancy and cancer. There was little on what are still termed 'benign'* gynaecological conditions. The World Health Organization states that 'Early suspicion of endometriosis is a key factor for early diagnosis, as endometriosis can often present symptoms that mimic other conditions and contribute to a diagnostic delay.'[3] Because it wasn't suspected, by the time I had been diagnosed it had already caused irreversible damage to my body. This situation is not uncommon, with the global average time to diagnosis seven to nine years. Some women wait much longer. A study of Arab women, for example, found that the average diagnostic delay time was 11.6 years, with almost a fifth of women waiting more than twenty years to be diagnosed.[4] In countries where healthcare resources are limited, women may have longer delays. This is because an accurate diagnosis depends on being able to visualise the endometrial cells through keyhole surgery. It's not as simple as just having a blood test or a scan to make a diagnosis.

Researchers have hypothesised that this global average of seven to nine years consists of two to three years of patients not coming forward to seek healthcare.[5] They attribute this to widespread societal norms that stigmatise talking about periods, and the belief that

---

*Benign gynaecological conditions are defined as those which are 'non-cancerous'. However, when the consequences can be infertility, chronic pain and multiple surgeries (to name just a few), I would argue that they are not benign, and are in fact very serious.

enduring pain is an integral part of being a woman. This means that women will often suffer in silence before reaching out for help. The next five to six years of diagnostic delays are thought to be due to poor healthcare experiences. Patients commonly describe having their symptoms dismissed, minimised or disbelieved by their doctors, with some feeling their doctors were gaslighting them – telling them 'it's all in your head' or 'this is normal'.

Endometriosis is a striking demonstration of testimonial injustice with individual women and other people who menstruate not being seen as credible sources of knowledge by their doctors. Consequently, they are not taken seriously. The intersection of sexism with other forms of oppression such as racism, transphobia, classism and ableism mean that some people are even less likely to be believed. Black women, for example, are almost half as likely to receive the correct diagnosis of endometriosis as white women, leading to poorer health outcomes.[6] It also shows how women are silenced – by being repeatedly dismissed by their doctors, they are deterred from speaking up, the form of self-censoring known as testimonial smothering that I described previously.

My day of being a patient at the Endometriosis UK scientific conference was enlightening in many ways, and crucially made me aware of just how much is unknown about the disease. Firstly, the uncertainty about whether Stage 1 disease (the mildest form) was the same disease process as Stage 4 (the most severe). And secondly, that guidelines to diagnose and treat endometriosis were mostly based on expert opinion, not robust evidence. This was because the *research simply didn't exist.* It was exasperating to hear this knowing that modern medicine had made so many advances in the last century, some seemingly miraculous, like eradicating smallpox. But we didn't even know what caused endometriosis, a condition that affected 1 in 10 cis women around the world, let alone know how to treat it effectively. I dare not even think about the prospect of a cure.

That was the day I became aware of a significant gap in our collective medical knowledge, one that continues to have personal implications for me. I still have questions that remain unanswered, a few of which I list on the next page.

- Why did I get endometriosis – was it my genes, or was it something about the environment that I grew up in that made it more likely?
- Are there other, less invasive, methods of diagnosing it than surgery?
- How exactly does endometriosis affect fertility? Could my fertility doctors have done something different? (In other words, could I have been a biological mother?)
- I am on a combination of hormones now until I reach menopause, which have side effects. Is there a better way of treating the condition?
- When will there be a cure?
- When I reach menopause, will it be safe for me to have hormone replacement therapy, should I need it?

Endometriosis is a devastating disease that we know little about. It has huge costs not only to individuals, but to society. It's been estimated that period pain causes up to a third of girls and young women to regularly miss days of school or university, and an estimated 600 million working days are lost to it in the United States.[7] This makes it even more astonishing that more investment has not been made into researching this disease.

In her series of essays, 'Painful Realities', medical historian Jaipreet Virdi recounts the history of endometriosis, showing how dysmenorrhoea (painful periods) have been regarded as a problem for a very long time.[8] Four thousand years ago, they were discussed in the *Kahun Gynaecological Papyrus*, the oldest known Egyptian medical textbook, thought to be dated to 1900 BCE. In 1860, surgeons saw endometrial cells existing outside of the womb in other parts of the body, but didn't know why they were there. Endometriosis was named in 1921 by John Albert Sampson, a surgeon working in Albany, New York.

So why do we still know so little about it? We may get some clues from how women with endometriosis have been historically treated by the medical profession, as individuals and as a group.

In 1948, influential American gynaecologist Joe Vincent Meigs gave a public lecture about endometriosis.[9] He announced that this was a disease mainly seen in wealthy women who delayed marriage and childbearing due to having careers. He advised his fellow doctors to withhold contraception from such women, for their own good. This attitude smacks of paternalism and victim-blaming. It also meant that endometriosis started to be seen more as a white, affluent woman's disease, leading to its delayed diagnosis in Black women and poor women.[10] Journalist Rachel E. Gross wrote that it 'is no surprise' that this 'blaming women for their own illness coincided with the rise of first-wave feminism and burgeoning suffrage movement in Europe'.[11] She noted that such attitudes, even when discredited, persisted, citing medical textbooks that still termed endometriosis a 'career women's disease' in the 1980s.

Even now, women are blamed for their illness. In an article by Sarah Graham, author of *Rebel Bodies: A Guide to the Gender Health Gap Revolution*, a woman reported that she was treated as though having endometriosis was 'a character flaw'.[12] Patients are also viewed as being malingerers, exaggerating their symptoms for attention.[13] Paternalistic attitudes from doctors are still common. Patients recount how doctors have advised them to get pregnant as this would relieve their symptoms – never mind that they may not be ready to have a baby, and that this would be a temporary solution as the symptoms would return after pregnancy.[14] Other women report being denied radical surgery such as hysterectomies, in order to preserve their capacity to bear a child. Such doctors have assumed a woman will regret having her womb taken out as she gets older – assuming fertility is more important to her than symptom control and quality of life.

As well as demonstrating the effect of testimonial injustice on individual patients, endometriosis shows how it affects large groups of patients. Millions of women, girls and other people who menstruate have had their testimonies of suffering systematically downgraded over centuries. The dismissal of their concerns has silenced them, making painful periods less of a priority than other conditions, and led to the gaps in knowledge we see today. And this is still happening where, despite the creation of specialist research centres like the Endometriosis CaRe Oxford, there is still an under-investment in conditions that affect women's quality of life. The National Institutes of Health, the largest source of medical research funding in the US, allocated $16 million to endometriosis in 2022. This is a minuscule 0.038 per cent of their budget, despite estimates that 11 per cent of women in the US have the disease. Researchers calculated that this worked out as $2.00 per patient per year, in comparison to diabetes which was allocated $31.30 per woman per year.[15] A further analysis in the US found that conditions which mainly affect men are significantly overfunded, at the expense of those mainly affecting women, which are underfunded.[16] In the UK, a health research gender gap has been reported, where despite a third of women experiencing a reproductive or gynaecological problem in their lifetime, less than 2.5 per cent of publicly funded research is allocated to this field.[17]

The lack of focus on endometriosis and other 'women's health' issues points to the history of Western medicine. Doctors and scientists have traditionally been male and white, and they have reflected societal views over time that say that a woman's role in society is to be a homemaker and to bear children. The knowledge these white male scientists have produced has reinforced restrictive gender norms and been used to further subjugate women. Those who have not conformed have been blamed and shamed for conditions affecting them. This highlights the inherent subjectivity of science, despite its claims of objectivity – scientists have been swayed by prevailing sexist attitudes.

In her 2022 book, *Vagina Obscura: An Anatomical Voyage*, Rachel E. Gross takes the reader on a trip through the female reproductive system, organ by organ, to show how the devaluing of women's concerns and bodies has led to gaps in medical knowledge.[18] A shocking example she gives is the history of the clitoris, whose true size and anatomy were not fully elucidated until the end of the twentieth century. She describes how Professor Helen O'Connell, a surgeon based at the University of Melbourne, focused her doctorate studies on clitoral anatomy after noticing that while much emphasis was placed on preserving male sexual pleasure after urological surgery, no thought was given to women's pleasure.[19] She discovered that the clitoris was not just a smaller version of a penis (as had been previously thought by the medical profession), but much larger and more complex, much of it not visible externally. Significantly, she reported that its main purpose was to give women sexual pleasure. This hadn't been considered before, as again women's sexual function had been ignored by the medical establishment. Gross reasons that in the past, many male scientists were either not interested in women's bodies, felt them inferior to a man's, or were embarrassed by them. This affected the knowledge they produced. She writes, 'The marginalization of women's bodies from science is largely due to the marginalization of women from science.'

In essence, women have been systemically under-researched, doubted, under-investigated and under-treated. Their ability as knowledge-producers has been discredited. The androcentric, racist and ableist roots of Western medicine have silenced the voices of women, particularly the most marginalised, and led to a lack of knowledge about their own bodies.

Here I feel it is important to say that women in all their diversity have fought back to not be silenced by the medical profession. The public conference I attended was run by Endometriosis UK, a large charity initially called the National Endometriosis Society. This was founded by Ailsa Irving, a Scottish civil servant.[20] She had been experiencing abdominal problems for many years and was diagnosed with endometriosis in the 1970s, requiring surgical treatment. In 1981, having suffered from the condition for more than fifteen years, she met another woman with endometriosis in hospital. Finding this experience to be 'a revelation', Irving placed an advert in a national newspaper to meet other women with the condition.[21] She received around forty responses and, on 1 March 1981, held the first meeting of the National Endometriosis Society in her house. The group gained coverage in the popular magazine *Good Housekeeping* and in 1982 it was registered as a charity. It provided peer support groups, information on endometriosis and advocacy. Now, as Endometriosis UK, it continues this vital role. In 2021–2022, it reported that it had run 276 support meetings, held webinars with experts, advised researchers and policymakers and ran awareness campaigns, among other activities that year.[22] Ailsa Irving died at the age of eighty-two on 17 November 2022, having left a legacy of hope to me and millions of people affected by endometriosis.

Patient activism – how patients have collectively fought to be heard – is a powerful force for positive change that I will be sharing more about in Chapter 6. When patient groups are silenced, doctors and researchers can be influential advocates. Many of the pioneers throughout the ages in 'women's health' have been women. But they too have been systematically marginalised and this continues to happen. When female and minoritised researchers are not heard, we all suffer. Without them, our collective medical knowledge will never be complete and will never fully reflect all human diversity. This silencing of minoritised researchers (and in turn minoritised communities) can happen at many different stages of the research process, from staff recruitment, to funding projects, to who carries out the research and who gets credit for it.

*

In April 2020, at the start of the COVID-19 pandemic, it was becoming increasingly clear that large numbers of people from racially minoritised communities in the UK were being hospitalised and dying. To investigate this at necessary speed, two leading research organisations jointly put out a funding call for research proposals. However, this caused considerable controversy when it was reported that the National Institute for Health and Care Research (NIHR) and UK Research and Innovation (UKRI) had awarded their £4.3 million to six projects, none of which were led by Black investigators. This was despite estimates that Black people were four times more likely to die from COVID-19 than white people. In response, ten Black women with research expertise published an open letter calling upon the UKRI to review and reform its systems and processes, so as not to perpetuate research inequity.[23] They wrote how affected Black communities must lead this response to COVID-19, not just be 'supportive voices within the research framework'. They implored research organisations to 'consider how their own practices and procedures might perpetuate inequality and voicelessness' emphasising that 'research funding and processes must be self-reflective about power and inequity'.

This self-reflection is sorely needed, not only at the funding stages, but throughout the research process. There is an abundance of evidence to show that racially minoritised researchers, and in particular Black researchers, face barriers at every stage of a career in academic research in the UK and US – from securing a post, getting funding for studies, to publishing research and getting it cited. These are all essential to be successful and gain promotion. Why does this matter? It matters because *who* does the research affects *what* is researched and therefore *what kind* of knowledge is produced. Without this, we cannot improve the health of Black and brown people. For me, this points to a systematic devaluation of their lives in research and medicine. This also happens at a global level, something we'll explore later.

When it comes to funding research, annual diversity data from the UKRI showed that racially minoritised researchers won fewer of the grants they applied for, with 13 per cent of Black applicants successful compared to 29 per cent of white applicants.[24] They were also less likely to get larger grants on average. Similar disparities have been seen in reports from other funders such as the NIHR[25] and in the US.[26] It's been suggested that this gap in funding is due to Black scientists being more likely to propose studies in community research, including health inequalities and patient focused interventions.[27] In contrast, funders show a preference for research topics that 'tend to have methodologies that are highly controlled with very precise outcomes' such as clinical trials and epidemiological studies. This was corroborated in a series of stakeholder workshops in the UK.[28] Participants reported that there was a gap in the evidence on the health of racially minoritised communities which was partially due to a lack of demand for this type of research from policymakers and leading medical journals. Stakeholders thought that more conventional medical funding bodies like the NIHR were less likely to fund such research, leaving it to charities and social science funding streams to fill the hole. These findings suggest that research rooted in communities (and led by researchers who may be from those communities) is not esteemed to the same degree as other types of research. When it comes to medical evidence, there is a hierarchy depending on what kind of knowledge has been produced and who has done the research.

Once research has been completed, it's essential to get the findings out to as many people as possible. This includes publishing work in academic journals, but this is less likely to happen to racially minoritised researchers. They are also less likely to be editors of those journals and less likely to have their studies cited by white researchers doing similar research.[29] These are all markers of a successful career in academia, so can have huge effects on promotion.

There have been many structural barriers reported for racially minoritised researchers, some of which I have witnessed in my academic career. These include a lack of role models, mentors, advice, and informal networks, all of which mean that these researchers know less about how to progress in the academic system. This happens right from the beginning of their careers as students. They may, for example, find that what they are taught does not reflect their culture or the contribution of people from their communities. I can see how having the work of people who look like you excluded from your curriculum may contribute to a sense of not belonging. For some, it may be too expensive to study, or they may feel encouraged by family to pursue professions where their earnings are more guaranteed (in contrast, salaries in research are often dependent on individual grants). Researchers and students of colour may experience racial prejudice, which can range from microaggressions to overt discrimination.[30]

All these barriers combine to reduce the number of racially minoritised scholars at the echelons of academia in the UK and US, leading to some depressing statistics. Science journal *Nature* reported that in 2021 there were only 160 Black professors out of 22,855 in the UK, of which 42 were Black women.[31] Bangladeshi and Pakistani professors were also under-represented. Among science professors, 88 per cent were white and 75 per cent male. In the US it was reported in 2021 that only 3 per cent of academic medical school professors were Black women and 1.7 per cent Black men.[32] This lack of diversity affects what types of research are done and the future pipeline of racially minoritised scholars. Dr Uché Blackstock, a medical doctor based in the US, wrote in 2020 about her experiences of academia and why she decided to leave after nine years, despite knowing her work was significant: 'I could no longer stand the lack of mentorship, promotion denial, and work environments embedded in racism and sexism.'[33] Dr Blackstock went on to found Advancing Health Equity in 2019, a company with the goal of partnering with healthcare organisations to dismantle racism in healthcare and to close the gap in racial health inequities. She warned that unless Black faculty and students are better supported by academic institutions, they will continue to leave.

The silencing of minoritised researchers also affects other groups for whom research gaps persist. Women, LGBTQ+ and disabled researchers are less likely to be successful in funding applications and more likely to experience prejudice.[34] For example, 30 per cent of LGBTQ+ people have thought about leaving employment in science, technology, engineering, mathematics, and medicine (STEMM) disciplines due to discrimination. This exclusionary behaviour was particularly experienced by trans and non-binary people.[35] Women report a lack of support, mentoring and encouragement to apply for funding. They also tend to be given more teaching duties, leaving less time to conduct their own research. Women are more likely to have pastoral roles, tending to student welfare, reflecting gender norms which say that women are better at care-taking. Taking maternity leave and carer's leave can slow their career progression. It is also common for grant application deadlines to fall shortly after school holidays such as in early January, which has more impact on women who may have had more family commitments over Christmas. They may also be less able to travel to conferences or attend work-related social events, reducing their opportunities to network.[36]

Disabled researchers report facing numerous difficulties with inflexible grant application processes, meaning they don't get the funding they need. Career progression may also be impacted by medical leave. Despite the Equality Act 2010 saying that employers have a legal duty to provide reasonable adjustments, this is often not done. Disabled researchers may also be less able to travel to conferences or for fieldwork.[37]

Women and minoritised scientists become used to having their credibility questioned, requiring them to work harder to be seen as equally competent to their peers. Senior figures in their departments may be more likely to hire people that look like them, which may exclude others. They may also be expected to spend more time on equality and diversity initiatives or student mentoring, which may take time away from applying for research grants.[38] A recent report from Oxford University looking at barriers to securing research funding in the UK summarises this issue well: 'A growing body of evidence underscores that academia is not a meritocracy. In academia, as in the rest of society, systemic barriers remain to limit the success of researchers in many marginalised groups.'

The report recommends that a systematic and co-ordinated approach from funders and universities to ensure accountability is needed, which must be done with researchers from marginalised backgrounds. It suggests practical actions, such as monitoring the characteristics of successful applicants, addressing individual and institutional bias, demonstrating inclusive leadership and recognising the impact of structural inequalities on marginalised researchers. They also recommended making information on funding calls for grant applicants more accessible and flexible, increasing transparency of processes, providing adjustments for those requiring them and mentoring for marginalised researchers.[39]

It's vital that this happens because when minoritised researchers are silenced, it profoundly affects what conditions are researched, whether the findings are valid, and whether they are relevant to the communities that have been researched. It also affects future minoritised researchers who may be discouraged by not seeing themselves represented in academic spaces. We will never reduce health inequities, unfair and avoidable systematic differences in health between groups without ensuring the voices of all researchers are valued. To improve our healthcare, organisations involved in research must recognise and work to address the impacts of racism, sexism, ableism, homophobia, transphobia and other forms of oppression on their staff and students. This will require investment, of time and resources, as well as a commitment to tackling prejudice embedded in their own organisational and institutional cultures.

I'm a minoritised researcher and my work has included studies looking at health inequities with regards to racism and sexism. As I'm also a doctor, my research questions have come directly from the patients I see every day in clinic and on the wards. I'm proud of the work that I've done and the collaborations I've built over the last fifteen years. But it's not always been straightforward. I have faced barriers such as those described in the evidence I've cited so far. This has been right from the start of my research career and it almost put me off pursuing more research.

*

One of the first research studies I ever conducted was on the topic of intimate partner violence experienced by women living with HIV.[40] This is recognised as being an important issue globally and one of the main drivers of HIV infection. It is known that women who have abusive partners are more likely to acquire HIV – this was because of non-consensual or coerced sex, or not being able to decide whether they can use condoms. Abusive men are more likely to have multiple sexual partners and be HIV-positive. Once women have HIV, they are more likely to experience violence from a partner, often being blamed for bringing HIV into the relationship, even when this may not be the case. Women have described their HIV status being used as a way to keep them from leaving the relationship, being told 'no one else will want you' or 'if you leave, I will tell your family you have HIV'.

Despite this well-established link, there was no research on the topic in the UK, which meant that this was an under-recognised issue. Historically, HIV research has often only looked at women's lives with regards to pregnancy. This has dehumanised them, seeing them only as potential vectors of the virus to their children and partners, rather than people in their own right. There have been few studies looking at their actual lives and this has left a large gap in our knowledge about how what they experience on a daily basis affects their health. This has made it harder to come up with policies that may improve the quality of their lives.

I first heard about the issue of intimate partner violence and HIV from a global health academic at a conference. Sitting together at the lecture, my colleagues and I resolved to find out what was happening to women attending our HIV clinic. By understanding this better, we could ask them about it and create local referral pathways to domestic violence agencies to provide support for them. We wrote a proposal and were awarded funding from a national HIV charity to carry out the study. This was a survey designed to ask our patients whether they had experienced intimate partner violence.

As is usual in NHS studies, before we could start, we had to get approval from an NHS Research Ethics Committee. These aim to 'protect the rights, safety, dignity and wellbeing of research participants'.[41] There is a long history of unethical research that has harmed and exploited non-consenting participants in Western medicine, so these are an important part of the research process. Committee members are volunteers and are a mix of research experts and lay members with an interest in health ethics. They are highly trained to scrutinise every research proposal for ethical implications. As a researcher, when I attend a panel, I expect my proposal to be thoroughly examined for potential faults, and I make sure I am as prepared as I can be to respond to queries. The research proposal should be improved by this rigorous process.

However, on this occasion, we were not expecting the proposal to have been rejected outright before we entered the room. The committee had decided that they didn't agree with the World Health Organization definition of intimate partner violence, as this included emotional and psychological abuse. They felt this was so common that if we asked about it, it would bias our results as many women would say they had experienced it. One committee member even asked us if we would 'label women as experiencing abuse if they had an argument with their partner' and whether 'isolated incidents of partner abuse were relevant'.

We were shocked by this decision as they had gone against internationally agreed definitions. Not only that, we felt that by blocking the research, this was going against the needs of women living with HIV. We spoke with several community members, women living with HIV who reiterated this – they wanted this hugely important issue in their lives to be recognised through research, realising that this was the way to get policymakers and clinicians to pay attention to what they were saying and work towards addressing it. We also discussed it with academic colleagues who had carried out similar surveys in other healthcare settings and had not faced this barrier.

We appealed and finally got the study passed through another ethics panel. We went on to survey almost 200 women attending our clinic. We found that more than half had experienced abuse from a partner in their lifetime, more than double the rates in the general population. The study was the first in the UK to look at intimate partner violence among women living with HIV and showed that it was a significant problem in their lives. It went on to be cited in several national guidelines and even now I am asked to advise on similar work in other countries. Because we started to fill this knowledge gap, national organisations now recommend that sexual health and HIV clinics have systems in place to safely ask women if they are experiencing partner violence and to support them if they are. This is in line with international World Health Organization guidelines that identify this as an important human rights issue and has been highly welcomed by women living with, or affected by, HIV.[42]

Of all the research I've contributed to since, I'm most proud of this study as I feel it was answering a question that was relevant to women living with HIV. For me, this is what research is about – exploring topics that matter to the people being researched. Otherwise, what's the point? We shouldn't carry out research just for the sake of it. More than a decade later, I still find it astonishing that it may have been blocked from going ahead, and that such knowledge, important for women living with HIV, may not have been produced. While this is likely to be a very unusual case, it made me consider that however well-trained ethics committees may be, they are still prone to bias, in this case, gender bias and possibly HIV stigma. Rightly, they hold power in deciding what research goes ahead, preventing potential harm, but they also decide what knowledge is produced. They can contribute to knowledge gaps and silencing in the research process.

Women living with HIV already knew that intimate partner violence was a significant issue faced by members of their community. They discussed this between themselves and had created their own strategies to address it. However, as the research evidence base in the UK didn't exist, it required an academic team to carry out the research to prove to other clinicians and policymakers what the women themselves already knew. Perhaps it shouldn't have taken the results of a research study to write guidance to support women experiencing abuse – perhaps the women should have been listened to as a group and the guidance written anyway?

For me this is also an example of what philosopher Kristie Dotson terms 'epistemic oppression.'[43] This refers to 'persistent epistemic exclusion that hinders one's contribution to knowledge production'. In this case a highly marginalised group (women living with HIV who are often Black or brown) have not been regarded as credible sources of knowledge at a systematic level, *even when the knowledge is about their own lives.* It took knowledge created by academic researchers (who have more authority than them in the medical establishment) for the issue to be taken seriously. Their ability as knowledge producers has been oppressed due to bias about their social identities.

Due to epistemic oppression, many groups of patients need advocates in academia to ensure research is done that serves their needs. But what happens when they, too, are silenced, as we almost were? As an all-female research group, with two members identifying as British Asian and one Black African, the feedback we received from the ethics committee was that we could not be trusted to do such sensitive research. They expected us to conduct research poorly in a way that would produce inaccurate results. Perhaps they overlooked our expertise, feeling that we didn't convey the type of authority they expected? I would argue that as most women living with HIV in the UK are Black or brown, we were better placed to do this research, as experienced HIV clinicians and academics of colour, than other researchers who may have better fit their expectations.

Since COVID-19 and the resurgence of the Black Lives Matter movement in 2020, many universities and research institutions have said they want to address how they have historically perpetuated health inequities in their own policies. By understanding their history, they can better appreciate how they have contributed to gaps in medical knowledge and amend their processes for the future.

*

The Wellcome Trust is a significant funder of research around the world and holds within its archive examples of medical knowledge both prioritised and neglected. I went to speak with a current employee, to see how change is happening today. The Wellcome Collection's café lives up to its name – a bright, welcoming space at the entrance of the museum located on Euston Road, one of the main arteries into London. Like this throughfare, it's hectic, with people meeting for coffee, or conducting Zoom meetings, or their heads buried in books. From the ceiling hang hundreds of transparent glass vessels of different shapes and colours, adding to its eclectic atmosphere. It's one of my favourite places in London to people-watch. I had arranged to meet Shomari Lewis-Wilson there on a damp morning in February. Lewis-Wilson is senior manager of the Wellcome Trust's Research Culture and Communities team and vice-chair of Wellcome's Race Equity Network. I first encountered him a few months earlier at the launch of the *Lancet* Series on racism, xenophobia, discrimination, and health, a collection of papers, one of which I had co-authored.[44] He had been invited to speak on a panel discussing how research funders can develop an anti-racist approach. I was struck by what he said and contacted him to find out more about what the Wellcome Trust was doing to progress health equity.

The Wellcome Trust is one of the largest medical research funders around the world with a vast investment portfolio of £37.8 billion as of September 2022.[45] It was founded in 1936 after the death of Sir Henry Wellcome, an American pharmaceutical entrepreneur. In 1880, together with business partner Silas Burroughs, Wellcome started a new company in London called Burroughs, Wellcome & Co. This revolutionised how medications were developed and sold. They introduced drugs in tablet form and, by using mass production methods and marketing directly to doctors, they operated throughout Britain and its empire. In accordance with his will, the Wellcome Trust was founded from the profits of the business to 'improve health by supporting scientific research and the study of medicine'. It has since funded thousands of researchers from around the world.

In recent years, the Wellcome Trust has been going through a very public evaluation of the ways in which it has historically operated and how this has impacted on health equity. In 2020, it committed to recognising and tackling structural racism within the organisation and in wider science and health research. This included an admission that it had *itself* perpetuated racism.[46] For example, in 2019–20, it had not allocated any funding awards to UK applicants identifying as Black or Black British. Success rates for white applicants were 14 per cent, remaining persistently higher compared to 8 per cent of non-white applicants.[47] The Trust made a pledge to become an anti-racist organisation by instigating a programme of work, which included an anti-racist toolkit for leaders, a set of anti-racist principles for staff, and training. It also launched a diversity, equity and inclusion strategy in 2021.[48] This aims for the trust, by 2031, to become a more inclusive employer and funder, and to promote more inclusive research design and practice.

However, an external evaluation of this strategy in 2022 showed that insufficient progress had been made and Wellcome remained an 'institutionally racist organisation'.[49] It highlighted that staff were still experiencing racial discrimination, there was a lack of people of colour in leadership positions and that many of the actions it had taken had not yet showed positive impact. It concluded that 'there has been insufficient action taken to allow this commitment to take root'.[50] In response to this disappointing evaluation of its progress, the Wellcome Trust has carried out several actions. These included setting up a targeted fund for marginalised researchers, conducting their own research into barriers faced by early career Black research-ers and committing to applying positive action principles to funding decisions and recruitment that will benefit minoritised applicants.[51]

I asked Lewis-Wilson about what made him feel hopeful that the work done so far will result in actual change at Wellcome, and what needs to happen for this to occur. He told me that in comparison to five years ago, progress had been made, saying, 'Looking back at the events tells a story of hard-working minoritised staff and allies from across the business doing their part to stand up for equity and justice, create narratives, convey needs and seize opportunities to push for change that has contributed to where Wellcome is now.' However, he continued with a note of caution about how the focus on this kind of work needs to endure, even with early successes. For this they 'need to figure out how to make more community, sustainable infrastructure and keep people talking to ensure that progress is not lost'. Here I think he really gets to the crux of the issue. In 2020, many organisations stated their intention to improve equity and inclusion, particularly around anti-racism, but was this just lip service? More than three years on, how many initiatives are still funded? How many resulted in positive change? With new economic and political pressures, how many organisations are still motivated to do this work and invest in it? Sustainability and constant self-evaluation are key.

I was also keen to understand more about the research culture within Wellcome, as I knew minoritised researchers can often feel excluded from their institution's cultures. Culture is a difficult thing to define. Scholar Sara Ahmed provides a useful explanation of institutional culture in her book *Complaint!*[52]

'When we talk about culture, we are not talking about something that is inert, already there, given, but actively being maintained through and in relationships. Sometimes by culture we might seem to be referencing some intangible thing; it exists, but it cannot be touched, given an exact description or value. What is intangible to some is tangible to others.'

An example of research culture being 'intangible to some' but 'tangible to others' can be seen in a study carried out by Banu Subramaniam and Mary Wyer in 1998.[53] They spoke to students and faculty at a scientific institution in the US, finding a culture that excluded women through 'unwritten rules'. Female academics described how these rules required them to learn to perform a set of behaviours and practices which showed they were serious about their scientific careers. They were expected to look and act in certain ways that were more acceptable to male faculty. These included not showing too much emotion, with crying frowned upon. When asked about these unwritten rules, the male faculty initially denied their existence (the rules were intangible to them, while being very tangible to their female colleagues). Later they went on to admit that they existed, but claimed they weren't prescriptive – they believed these rules were a choice, while the women felt they were a mandate.

I asked Lewis-Wilson about his vision for a more inclusive research culture at Wellcome and beyond. He said that, 'People and health research benefit from thriving research cultures and communities.' He stated his intent to not purposely define a 'thriving research culture' so that this could be interpreted to a degree. However, he believed that fundamentally it should 'value openness, collaboration, ethics, equity, diversity, inclusion and justice'.

The Wellcome Trust is not only interrogating how its research role impacts equity, but also its museum and library branch, the Wellcome Collection. This exists because Henry Wellcome collected millions of medical artefacts from around the world, some of which are on display. In 2022, it closed its exhibition 'Medicine Man', about their founder, so curators could review its framing, shifting the focus from one man to the objects themselves and who created them. In a statement they said, 'Our founder, Henry Wellcome, owed much of his wealth and many items in his collection to colonialism, and our museum and library have enshrined racist systems of knowledge.'

It has recognised that Wellcome's 'kind of collecting relied on and fuelled a market for such items that was driven by colonial activities and open to exploitative trading. Many objects were taken out of their social and cultural context and used to sustain a narrative that assumed European superiority.'[54]

This book itself is a result of this emphasis on health equity at Wellcome. With the writer-development agency Spread the Word, the Wellcome Collection ran a scheme in 2021 supporting authors from minoritised backgrounds to write a book proposal on health and being human. I was fortunate to gain a place and benefited greatly from a bursary, which gave me time to write, mentoring and workshops. It took this book from an idea written in bullet points on a page of A4 paper to a fully formed proposal with sample chapters that I could send to agents and publishers.

I left my meeting with Shomari Lewis-Wilson feeling impressed with the Wellcome Trust's commitment to health equity. I am hopeful that long-lasting change will happen. But this will not happen unless minoritised voices invited to the table are also *heard* by those with the power in the organisation to agree these changes.

*

Silencing not only happens within research organisations, but on a much wider level. Knowledge gaps are created when world power hierarchies favour certain countries and people. There have been significant differences reported between the treatment and respect for researchers in the Global North and South, with those in the Global South going unheard. These are linked to the history of imperialism and colonialism and affect many practices of global health to this day. How do these hierarchies operate, how do they hinder knowledge production and how does this affect the health of communities in the Global South?

We saw the significance of global health during the COVID-19 pandemic, but before 2020 global health was little discussed beyond the people working in the field. Global health had suddenly become relevant to everyone. For those in the field, global health has been flourishing for the last few decades. With increasing globalisation and the interconnectedness of populations around the world, we face new challenges to our health as citizens of the world. As well as the rapid transmission of infectious diseases, these include the effects of climate change on migration patterns and the pervasive challenges of obesity and malnutrition. Global health has been defined as 'an area for study, research, and practice that places a priority on improving health and achieving health equity for all people worldwide'.[55] Despite this laudable goal of health equity, the field has been criticised for its inherent inequalities in prioritising the voices of academics and communities in the Global North and silencing those in the Global South.* This is encapsulated by Madhukar Pai, professor of epidemiology and global health in Montreal who wrote, 'In short, global health is firmly centered on those with power and privilege, and focused on their generosity and saviorism.'[56]

To better understand why the field has developed in this way, we need to take a look back to the roots of global health and its links to imperialism and colonialism. Global health emerged as a concept in the 1980s, originating from the disciplines of public health (the prevention of ill health focusing on populations) and international health (medicine in developing countries). These in turn came from older disciplines – hygiene medicine (practices minimising the spread of disease) and tropical medicine (diseases arising in the tropics).

During imperialism in the sixteenth and seventeenth centuries, European countries were colonising the rest of the world in an effort to extend their power and influence. When they arrived in regions new to them, the colonising forces started to encounter diseases and climates that they were unused to, causing illness among the troops. And so the discipline of 'tropical medicine' was born. The

---

*The division of countries in the Global North and South is not geographical, but based along economic and political lines. Those in the South are usually low or middle income and densely populated, often those that have been colonised in the past such as in Africa, Latin America and Asia. Countries in the Global North are generally high-income countries and include those in Europe, the US, Canada, Australia and New Zealand.

colonisers in turn inadvertently introduced new diseases to native peoples who didn't have natural immunity to them. This had devastating consequences. Smallpox was introduced to Mexico by Spanish colonisers in 1519 and killed between 5 to 8 million people in 1520. Along with smallpox, other viruses like measles and influenza killed an estimated 90 per cent of Native Americans between 1492 and 1650.[57] In retrospect, it is apparent that infectious diseases were more effective at overcoming native peoples than the military might of colonising nations.

With increasing trade between continents, diseases were able to spread, creating epidemics. In the nineteenth century there were several global cholera pandemics which killed thousands of people. These spread along trade routes from Asia to Europe. Concerned by this, in 1851 delegates from European countries met in Paris for the first International Sanitary Convention, aiming to create an international health policy to contain epidemics.

Colonising countries used their military forces to set up clinics in colonies and implement often harsh public health measures on native populations. Healthcare was seen as part of the colonising mission, civilising native populations through Western culture and medicine. European missionaries and doctors brought over new medicines and scientific frameworks that they thought were superior to those of indigenous healers, negating millennia of local knowledge. European colonial programmes combatted epidemics of sleep sickness, plague, malaria as well as cholera in Africa and Asia. This wasn't a selfless enterprise – their goal was to protect the health of European nations and to ensure that the native peoples were healthy enough to keep productive and working to benefit the colonisers.[58]

In his book *A History of Global Health*, historian Randall M. Packard explains the link between these European colonial programmes and global health today.[59] Early global health campaigns at the turn of the twentieth century replicated colonial programmes. These included efforts to eradicate yellow fever in Havana and Panama by William Crawford Gorgas. Packard writes how this was seen as a good thing – part of 'a progressive narrative of international public health in which medical science overcomes age-old diseases and opens up tropical lands to economic development'.

Packard emphasised key principles of these campaigns, which he believed became the model for international health, and consequently at the heart of global health in the twentieth century. These principles were that:

- Public health interventions were imposed by the colonisers without consulting and cooperating with the local populations.
- Colonial rule meant that public health interventions could be sanctioned by law and therefore through force.
- Native health knowledge was discredited and disregarded.
- Native populations were seen as being incapable of taking responsibility for their own health, leaving them dependent on the colonisers.
- The focus was narrowed on single diseases, rather than health in general.
- Methods did not address the social and economic determinants of health, such as poverty.

As Packard shows, the medical knowledge of those in the Global South was viewed as being inferior – native populations were treated like children who had to be forced into doing what was right to keep healthy. They weren't credited with their own agency to know what was best for them. They were expected to do this while enduring inhumane working conditions to ensure that the colonising countries could continue to strip their land of precious resources.

However, traditional indigenous medicines have been shown time and again to be hugely important in the development of more modern medicine and practices.[60] It is estimated at about 40 per cent of prescribed drugs today come from traditional medicines. A well-known example is aspirin (also known as acetylsalicylic acid), the precursor of which is found in the bark of willow trees. This was used as far back as 3,500 years ago by the Egyptians and the Sumerians in Mesopotamia to relieve pain and fevers. It was not until the mid-nineteenth century that acetylsalicylic acid was created in a laboratory and in 1899 distributed as aspirin by the Bayer pharmaceutical company. The Madagascar periwinkle, a small plant bearing pretty pink and white flowers, has had multiple medical uses for thousands of years in Mesopotamia, ancient India and China. Currently it is a source of vinblastine and vincristine, used as part of chemotherapy regimens to treat several cancers. Vaccination, in my opinion one of the greatest medical advances ever seen, comes from the practice of variolation. This is an ancient method of purposefully infecting healthy people with small amounts of pus from a smallpox sore. This resulted in them getting mildly ill and developing immunity to the disease. There are reports that this was done as long ago as 200 BCE in Asia and Africa. It was introduced to the US by an enslaved West African man named Onesiumus in the early eighteenth century, and to the UK by Lady Mary Wortley Montagu, who observed it in Turkey and inoculated her own child. At the end of the century, this knowledge was used by English physician Edward Jenner to create the smallpox vaccine and pave the way for the development of other vaccines. These have saved the lives of millions of people around the world.[61]

Despite this history, the promotion of health was seen as being part of the wider civilising mission in colonial and post-colonial lands. Founded in 1913, the International Health Commission was one of the most influential health organisations in the first half of the twentieth century. It was founded by John D. Rockefeller with the aim to promote sanitation and 'spread scientific knowledge'.[62] By 1951, when it closed down, it had run campaigns in eighty countries against hookworm, bilharzia, malaria and yellow fever. Significantly, the International Health Commission financed the creation of schools of tropical medicine and public health in the US and twenty-one other countries, funding the training of health professionals from developing countries. These include public health schools at the universities Johns Hopkins and Harvard and the London School of Hygiene and Tropical Medicine. These schools shared common ideas about how to improve the health of peoples living in colonial and postcolonial nations. They trained researchers from previously colonised countries, who took the public health practices they learnt back to their homes, replacing local practices. Packard describes how critics of such curricula complained that they were 'heavy on science and scientific methods for controlling disease, but contained little material on how to work with local populations'.[63]

This legacy meant that strategies invented to control diseases in colonial lands at the start of the twentieth century became integral to the practice of international health and applicable to non-colonial settings. They went on to be the building blocks of global health today, building blocks that promote the scientific knowledge of people in the Global North over the Global South and that are enforced, rather than enacted in partnership with local populations.

As the twentieth century progressed, international health developed. The World Health Organization, an agency of the United Nations, was founded in 1948, with responsibility for international public health. It continues to collect data on global health, set health standards and provide technical assistance to individual countries. The majority of its funding comes from member states. Later in the century, the World Bank* recognised there was economic value in having healthy populations and started to invest in international health. While I understand the importance of this, it is telling that the moral argument was not sufficient. There was also a proliferation of non-governmental organisations (NGOs) and private foundations created, including the Bill & Melinda Gates Foundation, Médecins Sans Frontières (Doctors Without Borders) and Partners in Health.

The main approach to global health has been providing medical interventions that treat or prevent specific health conditions. For example, vaccines, medications, vitamins, oral rehydration packs, contraception. These are simple, cost-effective and can be delivered quickly without the need for much involvement from local

---

*The World Bank is an international financial institution that provides loans and grants to governments in low- and middle-income countries. It was founded in 1944 and now has almost 200 member countries.

populations. It is also easy to measure their effectiveness through research trials, cementing them as evidence-based interventions. They do not require long-term investment and they work without having to address the complicated social and economic conditions that cause ill health. They are cost- and time-efficient. I have no doubt that these interventions are extremely valuable and have saved millions of lives. However, I do understand criticism of this approach, which argues that it is victim-blaming – global health continues to see local people as being part of the problem, not the solution. It goes against collaboration and continues to value medical knowledge from the Global North over that from the South.

Alternative models do exist, such as Partners in Health. These prioritise longer-term sustainability, building healthcare systems that address a broad range of health issues, as part of wider development efforts. This is done in collaboration with local people. They take account of the WHO definition of health which includes wellbeing, not just the absence of disease, and sees health as a human right. However, they are often seen as being too expensive on a global scale, requiring collaboration across different disciplines, and their efficacy is less measurable.

Packard concludes that global health is a combination of these two approaches, but there is still too much influence from colonial models at its origin. He writes, 'International health interventions retained a faith in scientific solutions, a limited understanding and valuation of local cultures, and an inability or unwillingness to address the structural conditions that underlay patterns of sickness and ill health around the globe.'[64]

It's important to understand that the origins of global health lie in colonialism and imperialism, as its legacies affect research done now and in the past. Colonialism wasn't just about taking land, it was a broader concept, which has led to long-lasting impacts even when countries have regained independence. In their book *Inflamed: Deep Medicine and the Anatomy of Injustice*, writers Raj Patel and Rupa Marya describe this concept of colonialism as being when 'one cosmology is extinguished and replaced with another. In that replacement, one set of interpretations about humans' place in the universe is supplanted. Patterns of identity, language, culture, work, relationship, territory, time, community, and care are transformed.'[65]

Philosopher Kristie Dotson has written about the epistemic side of colonialism, in which local knowledge disappears because it is seen as unsophisticated and uncivilised by the colonisers.[66] Their knowledge replaces it. This dismissal of local knowledge has occurred in global health at systematic levels. And it continues to this day with researchers in the Global North deemed to be more credible knowledge producers than those in the South whose research is regarded as less rigorous.

These power imbalances at a global level result in significant gaps in the knowledge about conditions that mainly affect peoples in the Global South. One example of this is the aptly named Neglected Tropical Diseases, a group of about twenty diseases such as dengue fever, lymphatic filariasis, trachoma and leishmaniasis.[67] They thrive in areas where basic infrastructure like clean water, sanitation and access to healthcare is limited. They can cause significant disability and people with these conditions may be unable to attend school or work, reinforcing the cycle of poverty. Despite affecting more than one billion people, a sixth of the world's population, Neglected Tropical Diseases have historically received less attention and funding than other diseases. Perhaps if these diseases were a problem in high-income countries, such as HIV for example, they would have got more attention. It's astonishing to me that their historical neglect has become so entrenched that it has become part of their name.

Most aspects of global health have been set by academics in the Global North. This includes who decides what should be researched, funding, authorship, publication, conference participation, and membership and leadership of decision-making boards. A Global Health 50/50 report, 'Power, Privilege and Priorities', published in 2020 found that 84 per cent of the headquarters of global health organisations were situated in Europe and the US.[68] A leader of a global health organisation is three times more likely to be male, four times more likely to be from a high-income country and thirteen times more likely to have been educated in a high-income country.[69]

While academics in the Global South experience a credibility deficit, those from academic institutions in the Global North may benefit from a credibility excess, finding it easier to get funding for research abroad, and their findings published.[70] This then becomes a cycle, as with each research study funded and published, their credibility gets a boost. They are not experts on local communities, but enjoy the recognition that their work gets, even if much of it has been carried out by local scientists. They may be indulging in what is known as 'helicopter' or 'parachute' research, where Global North scientists drop in to conduct research in the Global South with the help of locals. They then take the data away with them and publish the research without acknowledging their local collaborators. This is increasingly regarded as a continuation of colonialism. The cost of this is that research done on local Global South communities may not be relevant to them and may not lead to changes that improve their health. In other words, the research becomes meaningless to the people it is done on and meant to be for. The *Lancet* now rejects papers submitted with data from Africa that fails to acknowledge African researchers.[71]

Researchers from the Global South are further silenced through barriers in publishing their work in different ways. Publications are essential for getting results out to a broad audience and crucially for career progression. But editorial boards, who decide what is published, lack diversity, being more likely to be white and male. Language is also an issue – despite a recent increase in scientific publications from countries such as India and China, academic publications continue to be dominated by the English language.[72] It is estimated that while 10 per cent of the world's population speak English as their first language, a huge 69 per cent of academic publications are in English. As these have more impact and are cited more often, researchers are incentivised to publish in English. But this means local communities may not be able to read the findings. If journals could prioritise publishing work in multiple languages as well as English, this would be beneficial. Otherwise, we are losing important perspectives from around the world, which should be contributing to the global knowledge base. Many publications also charge readers to access their papers. To reach a wider audience, many academics will pay for 'open-access' publication so people can read the paper for free. But this cost is often thousands of US dollars and discriminates against authors from Global South countries who cannot afford to pay it.[73]

Researchers from the Global South are also often unable to participate in global academic culture, which makes it harder to network and collaborate. Many international conferences are held in the Global North and strict visa rules, as well as the cost of registration, travel and accommodation, exclude Global South scientists from attending them. This means that the people from countries most affected by a disease may be unable to access the academic spaces where the newest research is being presented. A recent example of this is the International AIDS Conference held in Montreal in 2022. This is the largest scientific event focusing on HIV and is held annually. However, many researchers from Africa and Asia reported that they could not get a visa to attend. For those who managed to overcome this hurdle, there were still problems. The most high-profile example was Winnie Byanyima, executive director of UNAIDS, who tweeted that she was almost refused boarding on a flight to Montreal from Geneva. 'I'm @ Geneva airport, at the gate, boarding pass in hand on my way to #unaids2022, I'm almost refused to board, all docs scrutinised over & over again, calls made... I board last. Hundreds of people in the South have been denied visas & won't attend #UNAIDS2022 Unjust, racist!'[74]

Byanyima is one of the most influential people in the HIV sector globally and has previously also led Oxfam, the global aid charity. I have had the privilege of meeting her in London and she is an impressive and inspiring woman who is passionate about reducing health inequalities. However, because she is a Black Ugandan woman, she faced racist profiling at the airport and was almost barred from travelling. Similarly, Tian Johnson, founder of the African Alliance for HIV Prevention, tweeted that he was refused boarding on a plane to Montreal, despite 'nearly 20 thousand dollars in VISA fees, biometric costs, travel back & forth, public fights for VISAs.'[75]

There was considerable outcry over these travel restrictions with many people citing racism as the cause. The decision to hold the conference in a high-income country like Canada, rather than one that is more affected by HIV, was also questioned. In response, the International AIDS Society has announced plans to rotate the in-person conference around the world so that each region gets the opportunity to host it, and to also ensure virtual attendance is possible.[76]

The legacies of colonialism and ongoing practices in global health means that knowledge produced in the Global North is privileged over that from the Global South. It is regarded as more rigorous than that from the Global South. To achieve equity in global health, we need to make sure that Global South researchers (and their communities) are no longer silenced. It is clear that systemic change is needed at all levels, to ensure the meaningful redistribution of power from the Global North to the South. It should no longer be about saviourism, but meaningful partnership. This will require a re-imagining of global health that may take time, but progress is slowly being made.

In recent years, there have been increasing calls for academic global health research to be decolonised. Decolonisation in its most literal meaning involves the removal of settlers from colonised lands. It can also refer to the work of identifying colonial systems, structures and relationships within different institutions and working to challenge those systems.

Academic Linda Tuhiwai Smith made a powerful case for this in her 1999 book *Decolonizing Methodologies: Research and Indigenous Peoples*, detailing how scientific research is regarded as being deeply entwined with European imperialism for indigenous peoples in colonised lands.[77] Decolonisation been applied to many disciplines outside of health. Many universities in Europe and the US, for example, have talked about decolonising their curricula. With this they aim to challenge historical representations of the white intellectual tradition seen as being not only superior to other forms of knowledge, but as universal – the only true form of knowledge. While this sounds radical, in practice for many this just means diversifying the reading lists by increasing the number of texts written by non-white academics in the curriculum.

Other ways to advance health equity in global health have been proposed. These include making partnerships based on equity, mutual respect and trust. Diverse stakeholders should be consulted and leadership should come from those who are best placed to lead. Durban-based clinical psychologist and associate professor Thirusha Naidu has written much on power and epistemic injustice in this sphere. She says, 'We in the Global South need to find validity and affirmation and confidence in our own voices.' She emphasises that this will lead to less of a reliance on the Global North.[78]

Investment should flow to where the work is actually done, and to researchers from these areas. This requires political will, but would ensure that Global South researchers have the capacity and infra-structure required to conduct impactful research. There also needs to be an emphasis on removing structural barriers to inclusivity, such as hostile visa policies that prevent people from Global South countries being able to participate in global health discourse. Efforts are being made to increase the involvement of patients and other under-represented groups in global health organisations.[79, 80] It's vital that representation is not just about one or two people from these groups on boards, but many, going beyond tokenism to truly listening to their views and valuing them.

While this work looks promising, I end this chapter with a note of caution. The work to decolonise global health so far has its critics, who believe too little is being done, and that what has been done has been superficial. In a piece for the *Lancet*, London School of Hygiene and Tropical Medicine academic Lioba A. Hirsch asks whether decolonisation of global health institutions is even possible, as they have been designed to maintain their power and white supremacy. They benefit from it. As she says, 'They cannot decolonise and keep their epistemic, political, and financial power.' She goes on to say that if they are serious, it will require 'a radical redistribution of funding away from high-income countries, a loss of epistemic and political authority, and a limitation to our power to intervene in low-income and middle-income countries'. She believes this is unlikely to happen.[81]

This points to an uncomfortable thread that runs throughout this book. For people who have been historically silenced to be truly heard, those who have benefited from their silence will need to give up some of their power. Whether they do this remains to be seen, but I hope this book provides a clarion call as to why this is essential to improve health equity. When minoritised researchers are silenced, they cannot research health conditions that predominantly affect their communities around the world. Without their work we will continue to miss vital components in our shared knowledge of ourselves as human beings – this makes it everyone's problem.

Summary: How minoritised researchers can be better heard

- For research institutions, funders and universities:
  - Better data to monitor the characteristics of successful applicants and students and to act on emerging disparities.
  - Addressing individual and institutional bias, through training and policies that reduce discrimination.
  - Developing an inclusive research culture through leadership.
  - Providing mentorship schemes and formal opportunities for networking for minoritised researchers.
  - Diversifying curricula and better valuing knowledge created by minoritised people.
  - Making the application processes for funding, students and promotion more accessible and transparent.

- For academic publishers:
  - Diversify editorial boards and peer reviewers.
  - Reduce or abolish open-access charges for authors in the Global South.
  - Consider publishing in multiple languages.
  - Introduce policies which mean that researchers in the Global South are given appropriate authorship when collaborating with Global North researchers.

- For organisers of international conferences:
  - Rotate the location so they are more accessible for researchers from around the world.
  - Offer more scholarships for Global South researchers.
  - Allow for virtual attendance for scientific sessions as well as dedicated online networking opportunities so people are not required to travel to take part.

- For global health organisations:
  - Invest in researchers in the Global South through funding, leadership and infrastructure.
  - Build collaboration between researchers in the Global North and South for equitable partnerships and developing mutual trust.
  - Let Global South researchers lead on research in their communities, including prioritising what to study, the methodology and how to interpret and communicate findings.
  - Ensure diverse patient representation in the development of all research.

5

Objective

What Counts as Medical Evidence

'Doctor, what would you do if you were me?' Harriet asked.

Dr Agyei sighed inwardly. This was always such a difficult question to answer. Firstly, how could she really know what it was like to be in Harriet's shoes? She knows what she would do, but it doesn't mean that's what's right for her patient. And secondly, this was one of those situations where although she explained the medical evidence available, the answer is not clear-cut.

Harriet had been registered at Dr Agyei's surgery for over fifteen years, but it was only in the last few years that she had needed much medical input. She thought ruefully about how since turning seventy, the diagnoses kept stacking up – first high blood pressure, then increased cholesterol, osteoporosis, a stomach ulcer and arthritis. With each condition, she was started on a new treatment. She was on so many tablets now, that she imagines herself rattling after she takes them.

Now aged seventy-three, this was the third time she'd seen Dr Agyei in the last three months. Harriet had been falling. Not very often and with no grave injuries, but enough to make her worried about what was going on. The last fall had really scared her. She'd got up to go to the toilet in the middle of the night as usual and the next thing she knew, she was lying on the floor of the bathroom with scrapes on her arms and large bruises blooming on her face from where she'd hit her chin on the edge of the bath. Harriet had always been an active woman but had started to lose her confidence. And the timing was awful as she had been planning a long-awaited trip abroad next year – a three-month cruise around the world with her wife and their best friends. Hopefully whatever this was wouldn't scupper their plans.

Dr Agyei had examined her and sent her for some tests including blood tests and a heart tracing. Everything came back normal. However, because Harriet said she sometimes felt dizzy when she stood up quickly, her doctor suggested that low blood pressure may be the cause of the falls. Dr Agyei proposed reducing or stopping her blood pressure treatment. Harriet was worried about this – her mother had died from a massive heart attack aged just sixty-eight, and she knew that this was something that ran in her family. Controlling her blood pressure had always been important to her as a way of preventing heart disease and strokes. She expressed her concerns to Dr Agyei who replied, 'This is a balance of risk. We need to think about the very real possibility of you having a serious injury from falling, especially with your thin bones, versus the chances of you having a heart attack.'

Dr Agyei explained that Harriet had a 20 per cent chance of having a heart attack in the next ten years, and stopping the blood pressure tablets may increase this. But if she fell and broke her hip, there was a chance she may not recover. Research showed that people aged over sixty-five who had a hip fracture were three times more likely to die in the following year than those who didn't. It was a dilemma and Harriet wasn't sure what to do. She didn't want to keep falling, but then she didn't want to have a heart attack either. She remembered how devastating it was to lose her mother so suddenly. She asked Dr Agyei for her opinion.

'I know this is a difficult decision. The problem is that we don't have the research evidence to tell us what to do. Our treatment guidelines are based on trials which tested the drugs on people who were younger than you and didn't have many other health conditions. So, they show the drugs are effective, but don't tell us what happens in older people, such as whether they get more side effects. We need to think about what works for you,' Dr Agyei said.

They deliberated further and eventually agreed to reduce the blood pressure medications for a short period and see what happened. Harriet would measure her blood pressure at home and record if she felt dizzy or fell. Dr Agyei would also refer Harriet to the falls clinic at the local hospital for further investigation, but warned her she may not get an appointment for several months. They both finished the consultation feeling as satisfied as they could be with their plan.

In this common scenario, Harriet and Dr Agyei have applied 'shared decision-making'. NHS England defines this as 'a collaborative process through which a clinician supports a patient to reach a decision about their treatment'.[1] This requires having a conversation which brings together 'the clinician's expertise, such as treatment options, evidence, risks and benefits' and 'what the patient knows best: their preferences, personal circumstances, goals, values and beliefs'. This is something I aim to do, and at a practical level it involves trying to understand what's important to a patient and giving them information in a way they can understand, so they can make informed decisions about their care. Where possible, I try to give out written materials or signpost patients to websites, taking into account their reading level and preferences regarding language. This has the added bonus of improving their health literacy, which gives them more agency.

This scenario also highlights how the medical evidence we work with is imperfect. The research showed that treating someone's blood pressure reduced their chances of having a heart attack – this was important to Harriet particularly because of her family history. But as Dr Agyei explained, the evidence came from drug trials where the trial participants are carefully selected. Participants tend to be young, male and white. Unlike those in a trial, patients in real life come from a variety of backgrounds, often have multiple medical conditions and take a variety of treatments. This means that it's not always possible for doctors to directly apply the results of these large trials to the individual who is sitting in front of them. This is not a rare situation – more than half of adults around the world aged over sixty have two or more chronic health conditions, so these clinical dilemmas occur on a daily basis in surgeries all over the globe.[2]

There are other constraints that impact the usefulness of the available evidence too. For some conditions, the research may not exist, or it may not clearly show a large effect that can help with decision-making. Most trials will follow up participants for five to ten years, so it can be difficult to talk about the long-term effects of a treatment. In my daily practice, I will often get asked about the long-term effects of HIV antiretroviral therapy. However, many of the drugs I routinely prescribe have been licensed for less than ten years, so this is hard to answer. When it comes to shared decision-making, it's vital that doctors appreciate these limitations in medical evidence, convey this to their patients and discuss any uncertainty. By being transparent about uncertainty we can also maintain trust with our patients.

Trust, as we've seen, is hugely important in the patient–doctor relationship. Surveys show that doctors are one of the most trusted professions in the world.[3] This is because doctors are expected to be up to date with scientific research and to make evidence-based recommendations. They use this to make patients feel better and this in turn reinforces trust. Doctors are also expected to maintain objectivity when giving advice. 'Objectivity' is a term that is widely used. But what exactly do we mean when we talk about it? The *Collins English Dictionary* says that to be objective is to base your opinions on facts rather than on your personal feelings.[4] Many professions require a degree of objectivity, a prominent example being a judge in court. They must weigh up all available evidence to come up with a legal judgement that may have life-changing impacts for the people involved. This must be done without bias. Professions like medicine that are seen to be highly objective are often deemed by the public as being more trustworthy.

Objectivity has long been a valuable tool of doctors and helped to establish medicine as a profession. Western medicine in its recognisable form today has its origins in the nineteenth century.[5] During this time, there was a proliferation of scientific advances, which helped to accelerate medical knowledge and practice. Traditional healing methods were abandoned for treatments tested using rigorous experiments. Standardised physical examinations, procedures and tools were developed; statistical analysis became more common. Germ theory started to be widely accepted and there was greater understanding of the pathological processes behind disease. Anaesthetics and antiseptic techniques were routinely introduced to make surgery safer. Medicine became more effective and more efficient.

Before this, doctors were in competition for custom with apothecaries and 'quacks' who also advertised their abilities to cure patients. To differentiate themselves and seem more skilled, doctors made use of scientific advances such as the stethoscope and microscope. Such tools helped to create diagnostic labels for diseases. This contributed towards a shift in the nineteenth century from using descriptive terms for illnesses to diseases. For example, 'consumption' was relabelled 'tuberculosis'. This was aided by the discovery under the microscope of the causative bacterium, *Mycobacterium tuberculosis* by Robert Koch in 1882.

To further differentiate themselves, doctors started to be regulated. In 1858, the Medical Act, An Act to Regulate the Qualifications of Practitioners in Medicine and Surgery was introduced in the UK. Before then, an 1841 census estimated that a third of all doctors in England were unqualified. At the same time, the General Medical Council was created to regulate doctors and ensure all were adequately trained. Doctors applied to join the first medical register in 1858.[6] The General Medical Council continues to this day – all practising doctors must have registration and a licence to practice and will be struck off the register if they do not meet set professional standards.*

This shift to medical practice based on experimental knowledge granted doctors intellectual authority and social power. It also contributed to paternalism in the medical profession – doctors (at this time always male) knew the science and therefore knew best. But as we've seen in the opening patient scenario, the science is not perfect and it may not answer our questions, as doctors or patients, fully. Why is this the case and what we can do to improve the evidence we use in medical practice for better decision-making?

---

*The first doctor to be removed from the GMC medical register for being unqualified was Richard Organ in 1860.[6]

Here I will introduce the established hierarchy of medical evidence, which privileges objective knowledge such as that based on statistics over other forms. This is important because doctors prefer to treat patients with conditions which have a large degree of objective evidence in their diagnosis and treatment – this is a concept called 'disease prestige' and it can affect how doctors listen to and prioritise patients. But is this evidence really objective? And how has it systematically discounted the voices of patients and minoritised people in its creation? I'll show how this harks back to historical notions of there being an 'ideal scientist' who produces unbiased and perfect data. The knowledge produced by 'others' – those who do not fit this image – even if produced with great precision, has not been regarded as objective and therefore valuable. But can any doctor or scientist ever be completely objective? It is clear that doctors value medical evidence differently depending on *what kind* of evidence it is and *who* has produced it. I believe that this has led to the prioritisation of knowledge that has failed to answer the questions we need it to in clinical practice. This is to the detriment of patients' health. But I think that by including a greater variety of people in its creation and by expanding the types of research we value and use, we can improve it.

*

It was a complete mystery. Why were so many more women dying of fever after childbirth in the doctor-led clinic at Vienna General Hospital, compared to its midwife-led clinic? It was 1847 and Dr Ignaz Semmelweis, a Hungarian obstetrician, was trying to work out what was going on.[7, 8]

This disparity in deaths was well known not only to hospital staff, but to the local community they served, where rumours circulated that the midwife-led clinic was safer. This resulted in women begging to be admitted to it. Some even preferred to take their chances and have a street birth rather than go to the doctor-led clinic. Semmelweis started to investigate by counting the deaths at each clinic over the previous few years. He found that in the doctor-led clinic where the deliveries were carried out by male physicians and medical students, 13–18 per cent (approximately one in six) of women died after childbirth due to 'childbed fever'. In contrast the other clinic, which admitted patients on alternate days to the doctor-led clinic and was staffed by female midwives and midwifery students, had a mortality rate of 2 per cent (1 in 50 women). This was a huge difference – it was no wonder that women tried to protect their health and that of their children by avoiding the doctor-led clinic.

Semmelweis surmised that the difference was likely to be due to an issue *in* the hospital, not outside, as the types of women admitted to each clinic seemed to be similar. Those admitted to the midwife-led clinic did not appear to be more robust or healthier. He came up with several hypotheses and used a process of elimination to try and rule them out one by one. Firstly, he looked at obstetric techniques, finding no difference; religious practices – again, no difference. Even overcrowding wasn't the cause, as the midwife-led unit, unsurprisingly, had more patients than the other. He came to the conclusion that the main difference was the people staffing the clinics, but he couldn't understand how this could have such an effect. Vienna General Hospital was one of the most prestigious teaching hospitals in Europe and as such, the hierarchy among the healthcare staff was entrenched. To even think that these deaths could be the fault of doctors was heresy.

Semmelweis' breakthrough came from a tragic accident. His friend Jakob Kolletschka was performing a post-mortem examination when he was accidently cut with a scalpel by a medical student. He developed a fever, became very sick and died. Semmelweis realised that there was a connection between the process that caused Kolletschka's death and that of the women dying after childbirth. He theorised that doctors carried 'cadaverous particles', substances from the dead bodies, on their hands, and these contaminated patients causing their deaths. Midwives did not carry out autopsies and so did not carry these particles. He suggested that the doctors and medical students wash their hands with a solution of chlorinated lime to get rid of these particles. And it worked! Two months later, there were no deaths in the doctor-led clinic.

Despite his success, Semmelweis was not popular with his medical colleagues. The medical profession prided itself on being more enlightened than the traditional healers of the time. They viewed themselves as being 'divinely blessed' and were outraged by the notion that they had caused the deaths of their patients. *How dare Semmelweis, a junior physician, suggest this? Did he not respect his elders?* Historians have also proposed that xenophobia played a part in their attitudes towards him as he was from Hungary, a country looked down upon by many Austrians at the time as being less civilised.

Although Semmelweis did not know what the substance in the 'cadaverous particles' was, he had discovered that handwashing was protective. We now know that these particles were likely to be bacteria, and that the women and Kolletschka died from sepsis. This was several years before germ theory* was established and well before Robert Koch identified a bacterium under the microscope. Because of this, Semmelweis could not come up with an acceptable theory of how handwashing prevented childbed fever and so his intervention was rejected by most of the medical community. He could not elaborate on what these 'cadaverous particles' were. His colleagues, along with much of the medical profession at the time, believed in the miasma theory of illness. This blamed illness on a foul smelling, poisonous form of air known as 'night air', which was released from decomposing matter. Diseases were not passed on between individuals, but by vapours which came from unclean water and unhygienic conditions. They also objected to washing their hands before seeing each patient – it was too time-consuming and would require new facilities to be built, with sinks and running water.

Semmelweis' position at the Vienna General Hospital was not renewed in 1849 and, feeling betrayed by this, he moved back to Budapest where he became the lead for obstetrics in 1851. While there he instigated regimens of handwashing, and as in Vienna,

---

*Germ theory says that germs such as bacteria, viruses and fungi can cause disease. It gained prominence in the latter half of the nineteenth century and continues to be accepted today.

maternal mortality rates from childbed fever decreased dramatically. Despite encouragement by allies to do so earlier, he finally wrote a book of his findings in 1861 – *The Etiology, Concept, and Prophylaxis of Childbed Fever.* It was published fourteen years after his discovery. Perhaps if he had taken the time to write it sooner, he may have convinced more of his colleagues to take his ideas seriously.

His findings continued to be rejected by the medical establishment, and Semmelweis became increasingly frustrated. He started to write letters denigrating his colleagues and even accusing them of murder. For example, 'You, Herr Professor, have been a partner in this massacre.' This did not work in his favour. Semmelweis became further isolated and took up drinking. His behaviour became unpredictable and chaotic, and he was admitted to a public asylum. Within two weeks he died, at the age of forty-seven, from septicaemia. He'd been beaten by guards and sustained a small wound, which was probably the route of his infection. Ironically, he died from the very condition that he had protected women from.

It was not until several decades after his death that Semmelweis got the vindication he so desired and deserved in life. Germ theory started to be more widely accepted due to the work of Pasteur, Koch and Lister. Louis Pasteur was a French microbiologist who through his experiments in the 1860s showed that fermentation and putrefaction were caused by organisms (or germs) in the air. Robert Koch was a German physician who identified the bacterium *bacillus anthracis* under the microscope and linked it to the disease anthrax in 1876. He went on to identify the bacteria that caused cholera and tuberculosis. Joseph Lister was a British surgeon who was influenced by Pasteur. He introduced antiseptic techniques in surgery such as handwashing, clean gloves and the washing of instruments, which revolutionised the safety of the field. His first antiseptic surgery was carried out the same month Semmelweis received his fatal beating.

Semmelweis was the first-known doctor to demonstrate through experimentation that handwashing could prevent infections. He was valorised after his death, being called 'the saviour of mothers' and the 'father of infection control'. He has been commemorated in several ways, including a postage stamp in his honour on the hundredth anniversary of his death, and the Budapest medical school where he taught was renamed after him. I'm embarrassed to say I hadn't heard of him until researching this book, which feels like a significant omission in my medical education. Coincidently I came across a statue of him at work, which I'd passed on many occasions over the years, and not seen. He has also been made the subject of a play, *Dr Semmelweis*, which I was fortunate to see in London.

Semmelweis is an example of a doctor who was unheard and dismissed by his colleagues. Despite probably saving the lives of thousands of women in his lifetime, he was not recognised as being a credible source of knowledge. The kind of medical evidence he produced through experimentation and observation (known as empirical evidence) was not backed up by theory, a form of evidence that was more highly valued at the time. The medical profession chose to ignore the success of his intervention, preferring to remain wilfully ignorant, rather than trying something simple that could save lives.

I think Semmelweis' story is heartbreaking, but even more tragic are the needless deaths of thousands of women because the rest of the medical profession didn't trust his evidence. In the play, they are powerfully spotlighted throughout, frequently appearing as ghosts on stage to remind the audience of their fate. In the play's programme, there is an essay by historian Elinor Cleghorn, who describes how these women were blamed for their own deaths. She says that their bodies were regarded as defective and unknowable and quotes obstetrician Nathanial Hulme who wrote that it was 'women's tendency to "corrupt" their blood during pregnancy, by failing to police their behaviours, emotions, thoughts and diets' which caused childbed fever.[9] The play ends focusing on the women who died, concluding that it was because they were 'the voiceless' and 'the uncounted', that it took such a long time to find out the cause of childbed fever. This feels particularly poignant when we look at current maternal mortality rates, which continue to show how certain women remain unheard and discounted – those in the Global South, Black and brown women in the Global North – who are more likely to die from pregnancy-related conditions than other women.

The story of Dr Semmelweis is important as it highlights how differently types of medical evidence have been valued by doctors for centuries.[10] This hierarchy continues today and means that our knowledge base remains inadequate.

*

The dominant model of medical practice in the last thirty years is 'evidence-based medicine', a term first coined in 1991 by a group at McMaster University in Ontario who claimed to be introducing a 'new paradigm of medical practice'.* It refers to a healthcare practice 'that is based on integrating knowledge gained from the best available research evidence, clinical expertise, and patients' values and circumstances'.[14] I can imagine that it may seem strange to read this. If medical decisions were not based on evidence before this, then what were they based on?

Clinical decision-making was based on tradition (how we have always done things), anecdote (this worked when I used it in a similar patient), expert opinion (I will do what the eminent professor in my field recommends) and hypothesising from basic science (this works in animals or in the lab, and it's likely to work in humans). Evidence-based medicine replaced this with a greater reliance on up-to-date research, combining this with clinical expertise and patient perspective. When first proposed, its supporters emphasised that it was about making decisions on the best available evidence, not telling clinicians and patients what to do. At its heart is the hierarchy of evidence, which places objective data at its pinnacle.[15]

I first learnt about the hierarchy of medical evidence in university

---

* Before 1991, pockets of evidence-based practice did exist and some were patient-led. One of these includes the book *Our Bodies, Ourselves* written by the Boston Women's Health Collective, first published in 1970.[11] This groundbreaking book aimed to empower women to make decisions about their health by giving them information about their bodies. As part of this feminist collective, twelve women wrote about topics ranging from abortion to postnatal depression, evaluating available evidence and combining this with personal narratives. It has been read by thousands of women and has been included in the Library of Congress exhibition 'Books that Shaped America'. The last revision was published in 2011.[12, 13]

in the late 1990s when developing skills in understanding and assessing research.[16] This was first described by the Canadian task force on the Periodic Health Examination in 1979. While writing recommendations to prevent ill health, they developed a system of rating evidence. Since then, more than eighty hierarchies of evidence have been created. The hierarchy has often been displayed as a pyramid, with the 'strongest' evidence at the top and 'weakest' at the bottom. The strongest evidence is thought to be the least biased, and therefore the most objective and valid.[17] Often this is determined by the design of the study.

At the bottom of the hierarchy are:

- Laboratory or animal studies, which are seen as weak as they do not include humans.
- 'Expert opinion pieces' such as editorials, which are seen to be subjective.
- Case reports/case-series describing the clinical course of individual patients, which are not regarded as scientifically rigorous as they are not experimental.*

As you climb the hierarchy you find observational experimental studies, such as case-control and cohort studies, where researchers choose groups of people with defined characteristics and monitor them over a period of time. Statistical methods are then used to answer research questions.

Above these are randomised controlled trials (RCTs), deemed to be the gold standard of study design, as they are regarded as the most objective. This is where people are randomly assigned into different groups. One group receives an intervention such as an

---

*While the evidence at the bottom of the hierarchy is deemed the weakest, it can still be useful and herald the need for more research. For example, the start of the AIDS epidemic in 1981 was marked by the publication of case-series. Doctors in different cities in the US reported clusters of young gay men who presented with rare pneumonias and cancers related to unexplained immune deficiency. This made people take notice that something unusual was happening.

experimental drug, and the other group is the control (they may receive a standard drug or a placebo). They are followed up over a period of time and at the end the researchers analyse whether the outcome of the groups is different, to answer questions like – 'Is [the experimental drug] as good as or better than [the standard drug]?' These trials are often 'double-blind' which means that neither the study participant nor the person administering the drugs know which group the participant is in. The randomisation of the groups and making the trials double-blind reduces bias.

Right at the top of the hierarchy are systematic reviews and meta-analyses. These amalgamate and synthesise the evidence from numerous research studies to look for overall results. They are highly protocolised and are particularly useful when individual studies have inconclusive findings.

Since I was taught about the hierarchy of evidence pyramid, it has been superseded by another commonly used framework developed in 2000. Grading of Recommendations, Assessment, Development and Evaluations (GRADE) was created to assess evidence based on a number of factors in addition to study design. It has been used by more than one hundred organisations, including the World Health Organization and the National Institute of Clinical Excellence in the UK, to develop their guidance.

On a typical day, I make dozens of medical decisions based on evidence from thousands of research studies. To do this, best-practice guidelines are essential, as I would never have the time to read and evaluate every research study relevant to my medical practice. No doctor would. Best-practice guidelines are written by working groups who go through the rigorous process of evaluating available medical evidence and making recommendations based on this. These groups often include patients or lay representatives. I have been part of such guideline-writing groups and witnessed this process first hand – it is thorough and well thought out. Guidelines are a form of evidence-based medicine.

After its introduction in the 1990s, evidence-based medicine quickly began to be viewed as a success, making medical practice safer, more consistent and cost-effective. It promoted objective assessments of evidence, reducing individual doctor bias.[18] An early achievement was the British Thoracic Society's guidelines on asthma, which were developed using evidence-based medicine principles. This led to a decrease in asthma deaths and ill health due to recommendations in medication dosing and approach to individual patients. Infrastructure to support clinicians in practising evidence-based medicine was established, including setting standards for research, support for writing clinical practice guidelines, and the creation of the Cochrane Collaboration.[19] This is an independent, not-for-profit organisation which was founded in the UK and expanded rapidly worldwide, to provide freely accessible, high-quality reviews of medical evidence. More than 40,000 volunteers globally produce systematic reviews related to a wide range of medical treatments, which are stored in the Cochrane Library. Cochrane's motto is 'Trusted evidence. Informed decisions. Better health.' Resources were also created to teach doctors basic skills in assessing evidence, appraising its strength and applying the findings to their clinical practice.[20]

In 2013, the charity Sense About Science compiled a booklet of fifteen examples of how evidence-based practice has benefited clinical practice in the UK. These ranged from recommending keyhole surgery over open surgery for treatment for bowel cancer, to reducing the length of radiotherapy needed to treat breast cancer.[21] A notable example was the introduction of steroids to improve the survival of prematurely born babies. These babies died of respiratory distress syndrome as their lungs were not fully developed. A prominent example is Patrick Bouvier Kennedy, the son of Jackie and President John F. Kennedy, who was born at thirty-four weeks gestation and sadly died two days later of respiratory distress syndrome on 7 August 1963.[22] In 1972, a double-blind randomised controlled trial showed that an injection of steroids given to women going into premature labour reduced respiratory distress syndrome and saved lives. But guidelines were not changed until 1992, after a systematic review of the evidence showed this clearly. Now steroids are given routinely to women in preterm labour and babies rarely die of respiratory distress syndrome.

Evidence-based medicine is now seen as the norm in clinical practice. It's all I've known, having started medical school in 1998. I use best-practice guidelines on a daily basis at work and feel comfortable discussing their nuances with patients and colleagues. While evidence-based medicine has had many successes, it has also been criticised and calls have been made to improve it. Here are some common concerns.

For some medical issues, there are questions about whether we are producing the right kind of evidence. For example, in randomised controlled studies, researchers will decide the outcomes that they want to study, such as, 'Is this new drug better than the old drug?' Once the trial has been carried out, it may find that the new drug is marginally better on statistical analysis. But does this mean it provides clinical benefit: will the patient feel better? And are they looking at outcomes that matter to patients? For example, patients may prefer to investigate quality of life measurements, rather than a biomarker chosen by researchers.

Evidence-based medicine claims to use objective data, but is this always the case? Bias, at its most damaging, can lead to results that are misleading and dangerous. Unfortunately it's not possible to completely eliminate bias in research, but attempts are made to minimise it. In most scientific papers, researchers will discuss the potential sources of bias in their study. This can include which participants are selected, how data is collected, which statistical method is selected. Even in meta-analysis and systematic reviews, which are at the top of the hierarchy of medical evidence, there may be bias in the selection of studies chosen. Once the study has been completed, there is the possibility of publication bias. Academic medical journals are more likely to publish studies that produce positive findings, showing an intervention is effective, rather than those with negative findings that show that an intervention doesn't work. Researchers need to publish papers for their career progression, so may be less likely to submit studies with negative findings to journals. AllTrials is a global campaign advocating for all clinical trials to be registered and have their findings reported, whatever their results.[23] I was astonished to hear that there have also been cases of outright fraud where researchers have modified their statistical analysis to come out with positive results, just so that the paper is published.

Another significant source of bias is around external interests – who is funding the study? Do the researchers have a conflict of interest? If so, are they being transparent about it? One of the founders of the AllTrials campaign, scientist Ben Goldacre, has written extensively about these issues in his book *Bad Pharma*, arguing that pharmaceutical companies have too much influence in medical research, exaggerating the benefits of their products and causing potential harm to patients.[24]

Objectivity is important in medicine, because not only does it influence the available medical evidence base for clinical practice, but it affects how diseases and the patients who suffer from them are perceived by doctors. Objective medical evidence such as signs, test results and numerical data produced by quantitative research is valued more highly than subjective evidence that is self-reported by patients or comes from patient voice, like qualitative research. But for many diseases we may not have objective evidence. There may not be a diagnostic test, so doctors may have to rely on a patient's testimony, which is by its very nature subjective. This can include conditions such as long Covid and myalgic encephalomyelitis/chronic fatigue syndrome (ME/CFS), where diagnostic criteria are based on patient testimony.[25] This lack of objective evidence makes doctors more sceptical of people with these conditions and may affect how they treat them. If the doctor can find no 'proof' of a disease, such as a clinical sign (physical manifestations of disease that are found on examination), they are more likely to doubt the patient. Doctors may be less likely to prioritise patients with such diseases, finding them less worthy than others – this is a concept called 'disease prestige'.

Disease prestige was coined by researcher Dag Album and colleagues in 1991, when they noticed during fieldwork that doctors had implicit judgements about patients depending on what disease they had.[26] There seemed to be a hierarchy in how diseases were regarded. They surveyed Norwegian doctors, asking them to rank thirty-eight disease categories on a scale of 1 (lowest) to 9 (highest) according to the prestige that they believed most clinicians would award them. This survey was then repeated in 2002 and 2014 so the results could be compared over time.

The researchers found that over the twenty-five-year period, the most prestigious and the least prestigious diseases remained the same. The most prestigious were leukaemia, brain tumours and myocardial infarctions (heart attacks). The least prestigious were fibromyalgia, depression, anxiety and liver cirrhosis. From these results, they suggested that clinicians assess disease prestige on three factors: 1) specific characteristics of the disease, 2) the typical patient affected and 3) the type of treatment available. I've summarised this in the following table.

	Prestigious	Not prestigious
Type of disease	Develops suddenly Life-threatening Has clear objective diagnostic signs Affects the upper body – particularly the brain or heart	Chronic Few objective signs or diagnostic criteria Seen to be self-inflicted Not generally associated with a specific organ
Type of patient	Young Likely to recover Accepts clinician's diagnosis Whose treatment does not end in 'disfigurement, helplessness or other heavy burdens'	Older
Type of treatment	Leads to a speedy and effective recovery Requires an active intervention High-tech Reasonably risky	Few effective treatments

Leukaemia, a blood cancer which affects children and requires intensive chemotherapy, was ranked the most prestigious. Researchers felt that diseases where the clinician found it hard to understand the nature and extent of the patient's suffering were given less prestige. It's unsurprising to me that fibromyalgia has been ranked the lowest. This is a chronic condition where the most common symptom is pain all over the body. It has a severe impact on people's daily lives. There is no test for fibromyalgia, so diagnosis is based on a patient's symptoms. Multiple types of treatments are recommended, ranging from drugs to cognitive behavioural therapy to acupuncture, which may have varying results on relieving suffering. The causes of the condition are contested, with some doctors believing they are in the mind (psychosomatic) and others believing it is a disease of the muscles and bones.[27] Patients with fibromyalgia often report testimonial injustice with their accounts being dismissed by their doctors, and other negative healthcare experiences. Even when they get a diagnosis, they report that this can further stigmatise them and they are regarded as 'difficult' or 'heart-sink' patients.[28] Interestingly, the disease with the biggest change in prestige over the twenty-five years was stroke, which became more prestigious over time. This has coincided with the advent of effective time-dependent treatment such as clot-busting drugs, which make stroke care more dramatic and successful.

Album concluded that disease prestige shows that conditions can 'convey meanings which are not restricted to the "strictly medical" for patients and health care professionals'. Understanding this is important as it can affect decision-making. When objectivity is privileged, then a patient's testimony is often discounted. Patients with low-prestige diseases that have fewer objective criteria are more likely to experience a credibility deficit when interacting with their doctors.

Many diseases used to be medically unexplained, until scientists found their cause. Before this, they were often thought to be psychosomatic in nature.[29] Asthma as an example of this, now well understood as a condition where the tubes that carry air in and out of the body get inflamed, causing wheezing, shortness of breath and coughing. Asthma is no longer considered to be caused by the mind. There are now diagnostic tests and treatments for it. For a disease to gain prestige, the following needs to happen: an understanding of the pathological process causing the disease (why it happens); the development of tests for the disease (to diagnose it); and effective treatments. These are all objective measures. The less prestige a disease has, the less likely it is to be researched. This reinforces the gaps in collective knowledge about it and further marginalises patients with it.

So where do the critiques of evidence-based medicine leave it for the future?

Limitations to the evidence base mean that clinicians should not use evidence-based guidelines inflexibly – they must consider the individual patient. Many medical defence organisations which offer legal advice to doctors say that while guidelines can inform medical practice, they do not dictate it. Doctors are expected to use their knowledge and skills in the best interest of their patients. This may include not following guidance, but they must then be able to explain and justify their reasons. Being transparent about uncertainty can also help maintain trust in the patient–doctor relationship, as we saw earlier.

It is increasingly important for researchers to recruit a wider variety of participants into studies, to be more representative of the general population. Some now have specific recruitment targets, such as 50 per cent women.[30] Women in particular have been under-recruited historically in medical research – often excluded due to pregnancy or breastfeeding. This means that they are prescribed treatments that have not been tested on them. In many cases this may not have a clinical impact, but it's possible it may, due to the fact that women in many areas of the world live very different lives to men. There is increasing work being done to address this issue by researchers and drug regulatory organisations around the world.[31] This is also where real world evidence can be useful – data collected from patients once the intervention or drug has been licensed for general use.

In a paper published in 2014, 'Evidence-based medicine: a movement in crisis?', Oxford-based Professor Trish Greenhalgh and colleagues suggest ways to make evidence-based medicine more practical for the 'real world'. At the core of this is ensuring the focus is on the individual patient. They advise training doctors to be better at dealing with uncertainty and to develop shared decision-making skills. They call for a broader research agenda that considers the complexity of patients' lives, and favours research important to them. Evidence should be more 'user-friendly' – created and presented in ways that patients and doctors can understand and apply. The authors emphasise that more studies should be funded independently of pharmaceutical companies and that care must be taken to reduce the influence of organisations with a vested interest in the results.[32]

Evidence-based medicine is the predominant model of clinical practice used by doctors around the world. It contributes to making the medical profession seem more trustworthy due to its privileging of objective medical evidence. This type of evidence is quantitative – based on numerical measurements which are analysed using statistical techniques. However, you may have noticed that none of the study designs in the hierarchy of medical evidence includes patient voice as data. In fact, patient voice has been systematically downgraded as a source of medical evidence for a very long time, as it has been labelled as too subjective and biased. I believe this is an important factor in making our knowledge base imperfect. When the objective is given so much emphasis, we lose the subjective voice, which gives us real and essential insight into the day-to-day impact of ill health. Beyond this, the subjective cannot be avoided in totality, so why can't we embrace the helpful elements of it?

*

Historically patient voice has been an important component of medical evidence, but it has been erased from records. In his book *Maladies of Empire: How Colonialism, Slavery, and War Transformed Medicine*, historian Jim Downs looked at the origins of epidemiology: the study of how often diseases occur in different groups of people and why.[33] He explains that quantitative methods used today (such as numerical data collection and statistics) were developed during colonial times. This was because 'Slavery, imperialism, and war offered opportunities to study a large number of people at once'. There was also an urgency to this – infectious diseases such as cholera were rife and killing both colonisers and colonised people. The bureaucratic processes of colonialism, which involved copious amounts of record keeping, was useful for physicians, producing data that helped them understand how infectious diseases spread. However, this data was collected from non-consenting subjects including enslaved people, soldiers and Muslim pilgrims. They were counted and they were interviewed to find out about the disease symptoms, its incubation period and its clinical course. In this way, their testimonies were invaluable.

Initially physicians wrote down the names of people they spoke to, but over time these individuals became numbers and then graphs and statistics. Downs writes: 'They have become ghosts disappearing into the darkness of the archives and replaced with theories and statistics.' Downs's research shows how these quantitative methods, which claimed to be objective and apolitical, became an integral part of public health and modern medicine. However, they were founded on the erased, unrecognised contributions of non-consenting individuals. He concludes his book with, 'This scientific knowledge derived from the discarding and exploiting of human life is the basis of our ability to protect humanity from epidemics.' In essence, patient contributions to our knowledge of infectious diseases have been systematically expunged from the records, their voices silenced.

During the nineteenth century as the medical profession evolved into its current form, there was a significant development, which was what French philosopher Michel Foucault termed the 'medical gaze'. In his 1963 book *The Birth of the Clinic*, Foucault described how doctors adapt a patient's story to fit it into the biomedical model that they are trained in, and filter out the rest of the patient's story.[34] Biomedicine is a framework that says that patients suffer from diseases, which are a separate entity to the person who is suffering and their social context. The body is seen as a broken machine. Diseases follow a defined clinical course, reaching resolution or causing death, unless a doctor intervenes. The main task of doctors is to diagnose and treat the disease. The doctor remains a detached, neutral observer of the disease and the patient.

The biomedical approach is the dominant framework traditionally taught in Western medical schools and continues to be. Medical students learn facts about the body in sessions on anatomy, physiology, pharmacology, and then facts about diseases. During this time, they learn to become the detached observer, who is distant from the patient, holds the medical knowledge and therefore the power. Foucault was critiquing this approach, which he felt was more doctor- than patient-focused. Doctors dismissed what they thought wasn't significant in the patient's account, regardless of its importance to the patient. This paternalistic attitude affects how well doctors listen, makes it harder to communicate with the patient and show empathy. We know that the doctor–patient consultation is an interaction involving both individuals, so doctors cannot stay completely detached. By understanding that illness is not just a physical process but one that affects the individual from a psychological and existential point of view, doctors are better able to understand their role as 'healers' alleviating suffering, rather than just 'fixers'. This is beneficial for doctors who may get more satisfaction from their clinical practice, and for patients who would experience more holistic care.

The biomedical approach also devalues the voices of patients as sources of medical evidence (seen as 'too subjective') and privileges 'objective' evidence such as blood tests or results from research trials. As a consequence, philosophers Havi Carel and Ian James Kidd reason that all patients experience epistemic injustice, *because* they are patients and have a subjective view of illness. This is called 'pathocentric epistemic injustice' – patients are not seen as being credible sources of knowledge, despite living with the illness. Their testimonies are downgraded and even seen as suspect or irrelevant if they do not fit the 'typical' clinical presentation of an illness. They are seen as being too close to the illness to make objective judgements. Carel and Kidd suggest that this can be alleviated by training healthcare professionals to have a wider conception of illness than the biomedical framework, which means they can better value patient voice and lived experience.[35]

However, there is a form of research that views patient voice as an integral part of evidence. This is qualitative research, which aims to understand individuals' social reality including their attitudes, beliefs and motivations. Unlike quantitative research such as cohort, case-control and randomised control trials, which collect data in the form of numbers and analyse it using statistical methods, the data collected is non-numerical. Patients' realities are viewed as a rich source of information and collected using observation, or by speaking to them in interviews and focus groups. If quantitative studies ask 'how many?' or 'how much?', then qualitative studies ask 'why?' and 'how?' Clearly this is important, and it makes sense to me that to understand a research question, both quantitative and qualitative research methods are important. But qualitative methods have been undervalued in medical research for several decades. They are often misunderstood and discounted by many in the medical establishment because they lack objectivity.

In 2015 there was an international furore about this when the Qualitative Health Research Group, based at McGill University in Montreal, Canada tweeted a section of a rejection letter it received from the *British Medical Journal* (*BMJ*) to a qualitative study they had submitted for publication.[36] This is one of the most widely read general medical research journals globally. The letter said that 'qualitative studies are an extremely low priority for the *BMJ*', giving the reasons that they are not as widely read or cited as other research, and may not be interesting, or be of practical value, to their readers.

This caused considerable reaction culminating in an open letter from seventy-seven academics in ten countries.[37] They disagreed with the *British Medical Journal*, pointing out how in the *British Medical Journal*'s own 'top 20 influential papers of the last 20 years', three were qualitative in design. They acknowledged that the *British Medical Journal* was not alone among high-impact global journals to devalue qualitative research in this way, but stated that while some research questions are best answered by quantitative studies, some are not. They gave a long list of reasons why qualitative studies are useful. These included exploring how patients experience care, how practitioners think, and to help understand why clinical interventions that work in trials are not always effective in real life. They encouraged the *British Medical Journal* to develop a more pluralist (wide-ranging) approach that moved beyond a 'quantitative strong, qualitative weak' position, and to also consider publishing educational pieces that helped readers better understand qualitative research. Other researchers and clinicians also wrote to the *British Medical Journal* arguing that by relegating qualitative studies to specialist journals, it further marginalised qualitative research and meant that general audiences were less likely to come across it. They emphasised the relevance of such research to daily clinical practice and decision-making.

In response, the *British Medical Journal* stated that it did not prioritise qualitative research as such studies are 'usually exploratory by their very nature, and do not provide generalisable answers'. To accusations that this silenced patients, it replied that it sufficiently included patient perspective in the journal in other ways, including: asking submitting authors to explain how patients were involved in study design; having patients as peer-reviewers; and having alternative pieces that highlighted patient voice in the journal.[38] Needless to say, many researchers were not satisfied by this response and the debate continues in the medical academic sphere. Personally, I believe that qualitative research provides a crucial narrative that is often missing from the numbers given to us in statistical research. I have trained in qualitative and quantitative research methods, finding both to be academically rigorous and to produce findings that are relevant. By downgrading qualitative research, I believe we are downgrading patient voice.

To show how useful qualitative research can be, I give an example from the *British Medical Journal*'s 'top 20 influential papers of the last 20 years', by researcher Joe Kai, published in 1996.[39] This dealt with an issue that came up frequently for family doctors – communicating with the anxious parents of sick children. It aimed to identify what worries parents most when their children become unwell, and why. He spoke to ninety-five parents in Newcastle in interviews or in focus groups. They told him that they were most worried when their child developed a fever or a cough, as this may be a sign of a more serious illness like meningitis. They felt frustrated that they did not have the medical knowledge to assess how unwell their child was, understandably wanting to protect them from harm. To cope with this anxiety, they monitored their child closely and contacted their family doctor for advice. From this, Kai recommended that doctors must acknowledge and take seriously parents' worries. This would improve communication between the parents and the doctor, with both feeling more satisfied. This paper has been deemed influential because it has impacted GPs' clinical practice on a daily basis and is used to teach trainees. This kind of impact is not easily measurable, unlike the number of times one paper is cited in another.

Critics of qualitative research claim that it is not valid because it relies on subjective data collection and interpretation. Quantitative evidence is valued more highly because it is seen to be more objective. Despite the strengths of qualitative data, objectivity is more greatly esteemed in medicine. To understand why this is, we need to take a more in-depth look at what we mean when we talk about objectivity and how this links to notions of the 'ideal scientist.'

*

Doctors rely on a form of objectivity called 'scientific objectivity'. The *Stanford Encyclopedia of Philosophy* defines this as expressing 'the idea that scientific claims, methods, results – and scientists themselves – are not, or should not be, influenced by particular perspectives, value judgements, community bias or personal interests, to name a few relevant factors.' It emphasises that scientific objectivity is often considered to be 'an ideal for scientific inquiry, a good reason for valuing scientific knowledge, and the basis of the authority of science in society.'[40] In this way it demonstrates that objectivity is also a value, which makes science much respected by the general public. There are several common elements to what makes people believe science is objective.

Firstly, that for scientific claims to be objective it is said that they should describe faithfully facts about the world. These facts exist naturally and are ready to be discovered by scientists, who then analyse them and communicate them to the general public. In other words, science is the search for a neutral objective truth, which can be discovered by using the correct method. This is sometimes referred to as 'the view from nowhere' or zero-point epistemology.[41] However, when measuring or observing nature, the scientist's own perspective may influence how they interpret a fact. To explain this further, it's not just scientists that have their own perspectives of the world – we all do. Professor of neuroscience Anil Seth writes about the science of perception, which is 'how the brain interprets sensory information to bring forth objects, people and places'. He uses an example that I will share here: imagine you are looking at the sky on a beautiful summer's day, marvelling at its vivid blueness. Your friend is looking at it in wonder too, but are they seeing it in exactly the same shade of blue as you? Seth says this is probably not the case, writing, 'Just as we all differ on the outside, it's likely that our inner experiences differ too.'[42] When we use cameras to take a photo of the sky, we know that the image made will be distorted. What the camera sees is different to what we see with our eyes, which in turn may be different to what our friend sees. For scientific objectivity, it's necessary for scientists to bring together their perspectives of a fact, to come up with a consensus that everyone can use. They must also be prepared to change their minds if this consensus is road-tested and disproved. And so, the objective 'truth' changes as more evidence is created and the consensus shifts.

Secondly, there is the view that objective science is 'value-free' or free from personal biases and external influences. Historian David F. Noble has written of the notion of the 'ideal scientist' who has dedicated his life only to science and eschews concerns of the social world, such as politics. He ascribes the origin of the 'ideal scientist' in the West to have its roots in the Christian clerical tradition, with the 'ideal scientist' having monk-like qualities. The 'ideal scientist' was invariably a white man with social standing who didn't have to worry about everyday concerns such as housework or childcare.[43]

This concept has had a long-lasting impact on scientific culture. It has been called 'the culture of no culture' by anthropologist Sharon

Traweek. She wrote that science's claims to be objective, neutral and value-free, where the scientist stands detached from society, *is itself a culture* – one with unwritten rules that say that to be a good scientist, there is a certain way to act, and to be. This culture is tangible to those who do not fit the notions of the 'ideal scientist' – those of a different gender, ethnicity, class, ability or sexual orientation. For those that do benefit from this culture (white men), it is invisible to them – hence the term 'the culture of no culture'.[44]

Critics of this view of scientific objectivity say that it is impossible for science to be value-free. Subjective decisions made by scientists are inherent in the scientific method. A scientist's personal values can affect scientific findings at many different stages of research: when choosing what research question to investigate, how to collect data, how to assess the data and how to interpret the results. To make scientific claims more objective, scientists should endeavour to reduce the influence of their values at each stage of research. This includes lowering external interests in the research, such as politics or business, and being transparent if there are any conflicts. Virginia Woolf was one such critic of scientific objectivity, writing in 1938 in *Three Guineas* that, 'Science, it would seem, is not sexless; she is a man.'[45]

The idea that science produced by white men is more objective than that produced by others has been at the heart of modern Western science. It has marginalised knowledge produced by other groups and continues to do so. Social epidemiologist Professor Nancy Krieger stated 'Knowledge partial to – and especially born of – the disempowered, no matter how rigorous and precise, never seems as "objective" as the other kind.'[46] We have seen this in global health, where indigenous and local knowledge produced by researchers in the Global South is viewed as being less legitimate than that produced in the Global North. We have seen this in the practice of medicine where the paternal approach was deemed the best way. In their essay 'Medicine Is Not Gender-Neutral – She is Male', Kiki M. J. Lombarts and Abraham Verghese argue that 'Over time, the physician's bedside skills – including history taking, the physical examination, and the use of the clinical eye – began to seem less important than "objective" data', such as blood tests and scans. They emphasise that this objectivity has been regarded as a male trait. 'Female qualities' such as empathy, communication skills and nurturing were devalued.[47]

Critics of scientific objectivity say that the inherent biases that all scientists have should be acknowledged and even used to its advantage, to make science better. Science philosopher Sandra Harding coined the term 'strong objectivity' in her 2015 book *Objectivity and Diversity: Another Logic of Scientific Research.*[48] She theorised that scientific objectivity, whilst being an ideal, is weak as it is not value-neutral and researcher bias can never be fully removed. She felt that a researcher's life experiences affect every aspect of their world view and consequently their work. I think the androcentric roots of Western medicine that lead to gaps in medical knowledge about women supports this view – male scientists worked in a society that viewed women as inferior to men and their research findings were interpreted in ways to support this view.[49] Harding says that male researchers attempt to be neutral and do not realise that they are not. Instead, she advocates for dropping the pretence that it's possible for a scientist to be value-free and suggests embracing a strong objectivity that takes into account a researcher's positionality and reflecting on how it affects their research findings.

As part of my dissertation for my social epidemiology masters, I looked at rates of sexually transmitted infections among people of South Asian ethnicity in England.[50] I chose this subject as I knew there was a gap in the evidence on South Asian sexual health nationally and I wanted to develop quantitative research skills. I undertook a statistical analysis of data collected by the UK Health Security Agency from every specialist sexual health service in England. When I wrote up my findings, my supervisors were keen that I included a paragraph reflecting on my positionality as a South Asian sexual health doctor. At every stage of the research, I also made sure to reflect on how this may influence me and the work – such as not overstating the importance of a finding, because it was personally interesting to me. I think my positionality has also been an asset here, an example of 'strong objectivity'. Because of my background I chose to do the research – if I hadn't done it, no one else may have carried it out and the research gap may still exist. This process of self-reflection is regularly done in qualitative research, but rarely in quantitative. There are calls for this to change and I think this would be a good step forward. It would mean that when we read research, we can understand where the scientist is coming from, and how this may affect their methodology and interpretation of their findings.

We cannot avoid human messiness but there remains this 'myth of objectivity' within science, medicine and evidence. Subjective questions and information hold value, and while the objective holds importance, it shouldn't mean that we silence what the subjective can bring. As classificationist Melanie Feinberg shares, 'data is created, not found; and creating it well demands humanity, rather than objectivity'.[51, 52] Beyond this, perhaps what we deem to be objective medical evidence is not quite as objective as we first thought. This doesn't make it any less important. Instead, doctors need to understand its limitations and think about what else we can use to strengthen our knowledge base. Involving patient voices, and expanding into the subjective in evidence and research may seem like an unwieldy task, but it's already happening with excellent results.

*

Patient and public involvement improves research because it ensures that studies are relevant to patients – hearing this always makes me smile, as surely this should be the main goal of health research? It improves the way in which studies are carried out and helps get the results out to a wider range of people. It enhances participants' experiences of research, which may make them more likely to take part in future studies. This is hugely important: the record of unethical research globally has understandably put people off taking part – they do not trust the researchers not to harm them.

While patient and public involvement can occur in a variety of ways and at any stage of the process, a large review found that roles mainly included giving feedback on research that had already been designed, rather than fundamentally shaping the research.[53] Critics of current practice say that patient and public involvement is often seen as an optional extra or even tokenistic.[54] There have been calls for more meaningful patient and public involvement through approaches that take into account the power imbalances that exist between academics, clinicians and patients. When power is skewed towards clinicians and academics, there is a danger that this can negatively affect research in several ways – inappropriate research questions, unethical methodology, interpreting results in a way that reinforces inequalities and the exclusion of marginalised groups. Patient power in health research helps to reduce this risk. The movement for more meaningful patient and public involvement includes approaches such as co-production, priority-setting partnerships and community conversations.

'Co-production' is defined as a way of working together in equal partnership and for equal benefit. It is gaining prominence both in medical research and in policy areas. Lynn Laidlaw, a public and patient contributor to health research, introduced me to the work of the Co-production Collective based at University College London, which she is part of. On its website, this collective describes itself as a community 'where everyone is welcome'. It explains co-production as 'bringing together different forms of lived or living and learnt (personal and professional) knowledge, understanding and experience for better outcomes and mutual benefit'. It states four components of its approach:

1. Being Human: valuing diversity of knowledge, experience and perspective. Building mutually beneficial relationships based on honesty and trust.
2. Being inclusive: removing barriers to participation. Recognising people's strengths and supporting their development.
3. Bring transparent: addressing power imbalances and hierarchies. Sharing roles and responsibilities.
4. Being challenging: continuous reflection, learning and improvement. Embracing new ideas and ways of working.

This allows patients, researchers, clinicians and policymakers to work together as one team.

The Collective gathered evidence to create a resource highlighting the importance of co-production – they found it delivers outcomes that matter to patients, improves efficiency, enables capacity building, empowers people and works towards social justice. However, they caution that co-production is 'not a fix all' and may not always be the most appropriate research approach – it depends on the context.[55]

Laidlaw said to me, 'There is a phrase about co-production that "it's a state of being, not of doing", that resonates with me. It's essentially a values- and principles-led way of working that is mindful of power imbalances: the culture in which it operates is of prime importance. It's messy and emotional, requires reflexivity and is founded on relationships, collaboration and conversation.'

Laidlaw described being involved in co-production as a contributor to be hugely important to her. It meant a lot to have people believe in her as a patient researcher. She emphasised that it is a patient's right to be involved in research, and for them it's even more significant as they are personally invested - research into a person's condition can 'literally be life or death'. However, Laidlaw acknowledged it wasn't always easy to be a patient contributor/researcher and there were ways in which they could be better supported.

She shared some sage advice for researchers who want to work with patient contributors. This includes:

- Giving a realistic expectation of the time and work required.
- Providing compensation, training, supervision and opportunities to debrief.
- Changing research culture itself – to go from privileging publications, grants and citations as metrics of a successful researcher, to more highly valuing the so-called 'soft skills' of collaboration, dialogue and building relationships.

Another emerging approach to patient and public involvement are community conversations – a means to engage a large number of community members in dialogue about an issue. They have been used successfully in Southern Africa, developing community-led inter-ventions and solutions for issues related to HIV and gender-based violence. Rochelle Burgess, associate professor in global health at University College London, and colleagues have recently successfully used community conversations to inform the design of a large clinical trial in Nigeria. This aimed to reduce deaths among children under five. They held twelve community conversations with a total of 320 participants to explore their views on pneumonia in young children. They divided these participants into three smaller groups: younger women, older women and men. Conversations were facilitated by community researchers and included discussions and drawing activ-ities to make sure everyone could take part. From this, they identified issues that they used to adapt their clinical trial, such as factors that could affect its implementation. They noted how positively partici-pants engaged in the process – many said they valued the opportunity to express their views in a way they couldn't in the past. This was particularly true for the younger women aged between eighteen and thirty, who were in their own group and often felt silenced around men and older women. The researchers concluded that this process was beneficial for their trial but also for the community. Importantly, it provided 'a pathway to engage everyday citizens as experts in the processes of knowledge production in more meaningful ways'.[56]

The last approach to working with patients that I will mention here is priority-setting partnerships. These are initiatives to help patients, carers and clinicians work together to identify and prioritise areas of uncertainty in the evidence about a health condition. In the UK they are often facilitated by the James Lind Alliance, which was set up in 2004 with the aim of opening up conversations between clinicians and patients.* A health topic is chosen and through a

---

* James Lind was a Scottish naval surgeon in the eighteenth century who discovered that oranges and lemons were an effective treatment against scurvy, a deadly disease that killed sailors on long sea voyages. He did this by creating a clinical trial, allocating two soldiers into each arm of the trial and testing six different treatments for fourteen days. Oranges and lemons were the most effective, and we now know that this is because they contain vitamin C. Scurvy is caused by a deficiency of this.

facilitated multistage process, the group produces a final top ten list of jointly agreed research priorities. This list is made publicly available for researchers and funders to access.[57, 58] The first priority-setting partnership in the UK was completed in 2007 and looked at asthma. The top ten research priorities agreed upon included 'What are the key components of successful "self-management" for a person with asthma?' and 'What are the adverse effects associated with long-term use of different types of therapy in adults?' Since then, over one hundred priority-setting partnerships have been carried out in different areas of health. In this way, patients, clinicians and people affected by a disease have a say in what research is carried out. It works because it puts these different groups on an equal footing, excludes groups with a conflict of interest (such as drug companies) and is a transparent process.

Patient and public involvement in research is an evolving field and I have only skimmed the surface of what is being done around the world. I believe research needs to be useful and, where possible, helpful to the people that it involves. They need to see it has impact. I was struck by the title of a recent report, 'Why am I always being researched?' by Chicago Beyond, a funder of community work promoting youth equity in the US. These were words uttered by Jonte, a young man living in Chicago, in reaction to having taken part, like many of his community, in multiple research studies over the years. The report explains how despite millions of dollars being invested, 'the fruits of those studies have infrequently nourished the neighbourhoods where their seeds were planted'. In other words, communities did not feel the benefits of the research they were a part of. This has engendered a deep distrust between the community and the researchers, despite their good intentions.[59] Patients' voices must be at the heart of research right from the start and it should benefit them.

*

Objectivity has its place in medicine, but the privileging of it can silence patient voices. Doctors and researchers are at their best when they understand the limits of their own objectivity – like everyone in society, they hold their own inherent biases and prejudices. Reflecting on these and admitting they exist is a first step to tackling them. For me this includes accepting that being a doctor has affected my experiences of being a patient.

We should always consider whether we are taking up space that would be better filled by someone with more direct experience. When I first wrote about my experience of being denied pain relief in an essay for the medical journal the *Lancet*, I received generally very positive responses from patients and doctors for raising awareness of the issue. But a couple of patients asked on social media why it had taken a doctor to write about the common experience of being unheard, for this to be published. This is an important question. Why are patient experiences only validated when doctors experience them? And why are we more likely to be heard? This again points to notions of expertise – as doctors we are experts in medicine, but once again this devalues patients' expertise that comes from lived experience. By acknowledging that both forms of knowledge are important, we can improve not only research, but medicine as a whole.

Summary: How we can produce better medical evidence

- Increase the range of people conducting research to include minoritised scientists and people with lived experience.
- Involve patients and the public in research from inception and at every stage of the study.
- Better support people with lived experience when carrying out research.
- Improve research literacy by presenting it in formats that are easier for patients and doctors to understand.
- Work with communities to recruit more women, older people and those from minoritised groups into research studies.
- Train doctors to better understand the limitations of medical evidence, to communicate this to patients and deal with uncertainty.
- Academic journals, guideline writing groups, medical societies and research institutions need to place a higher value on research studies that aren't quantitative and use a greater range of data as medical evidence.
- Academic journals should publish more research with negative results.
- Ensure that there is a range of research funding sources apart from those provided by pharmaceutical companies and industries.
- Ensure conflicts of interest are correctly stated and prominently displayed whenever research findings are disseminated.

6

Roar

How Patients Fought to Get Heard

'I thought my life was over. I can't believe I'm sitting here now with Angel speaking to you, and we are OK. Better than OK, in fact! Life is good.'

Alice smiles and bounces Angel, her fittingly named daughter, on her lap. The baby looks at me, her deep brown eyes framed by long eyelashes. She blinks and then yawns, nuzzling her head into her mother's welcoming belly, her interest in her surroundings sated. I focus my attention onto her mother. She looks like a completely different woman to the one I met two years earlier, pregnant, having just been diagnosed with HIV.

Originally from France, Alice had moved to the UK four years previously, to be with her new husband. She was looking forward to starting their life together. When they'd met, he'd seemed charming and considerate, but once they were married, she saw a different side to him. He was controlling, deciding when she could go out, who she could see and how she could spend her money. She also discovered that he had a girlfriend and a young son whom he was providing for.

When Alice found out she was pregnant, he left her and moved in with his other family. This felt like a mixed blessing – she was finally free of him, but found herself unemployed, pregnant and alone. And then to top it all, the midwife told her that her antenatal bloods had shown she was HIV positive. By the time I met her in my HIV clinic, she was shell-shocked and desperate, scared for her own health and that of her unborn child. I remember trying to reassure her that it would get better, that we could help her, but I wasn't sure she believed me.

A lot had happened in the two years since then. She was started on HIV antiretroviral therapy, three different drugs combined into two tablets, to reduce the amount of virus in her body to undetectable levels. This prevented the HIV from weakening her immune system and she remained physically well during her pregnancy. It also meant that she could have a normal vaginal delivery, and she gave birth to Angel, who was HIV-negative.

During the pregnancy, she was seen regularly in antenatal clinic by our multidisciplinary team. This included a HIV specialist midwife, an obstetrician and me, a HIV doctor. We assessed her additional needs. A social worker filled out forms with her to ensure she was receiving the benefits she was entitled to and she was seen regularly by our inhouse psychologist. She agreed to be referred to a HIV peer support programme and was matched with a local mentor-mother. This was a woman living with HIV who was trained to provide peer support to other women with HIV. Having had children herself, she could share her lived experiences of HIV, pregnancy and motherhood with Alice, information that we in the clinical team could not provide. Crucially, she provided Alice with companionship, introducing her to a group of women living with HIV, who went on to become her friends. Each time I saw Alice in clinic, she seemed less anxious and more comfortable with speaking up.

Two years on, Alice and Angel are healthy and thriving. Alice is about to start a new job in IT, having completed a masters in the subject before she got married. She is now divorced and no longer in contact with her ex-husband. She tells me she is happily single, but has met a friend at church that she seems to spend a lot of time with, and who makes her smile whenever she mentions him. She exudes an air of quiet contentedness and seems upbeat about the future.

As I hand her a prescription and bid her farewell for six months until her next appointment, I reflect on how I have one of the best jobs in the world. I am lucky to work in HIV medicine at a time where effective treatment and services are available to provide holistic whole-person care – I witness people's lives changing for the better. It is a wonderful thing to tell a person who has been diagnosed and is in despair that things will improve for them. I can give them the gift of hope.

This has not always been the case. Until 1996, when combination therapy was discovered, HIV was a terminal condition. People with the virus were ostracised by society and neglected by governments tasked with their care. They had no choice but to speak up. That HIV became a treatable condition within fifteen years of the epidemic starting is testament to their work – thousands of activists, many living with HIV, who agitated for treatment, care and their human rights.

There is a long history of patients who have fought to be heard despite systematic silencing, and people with HIV/AIDS are a recent but significant example. They have changed medicine in a broader sense – influencing its language, how healthcare is delivered and the importance of addressing the structural and social determinants that affect peoples' health. They have also transformed how science is done – expanding ideas of who is deemed to have scientific expertise, who creates new knowledge and how clinical trials are run. Crucially, people living with HIV have held governments and industry to account, asking why some peoples' lives are treated as less valuable than others.

*

ACT UP Albany Action, Albany, New York State, 9 May 1988.

The video on YouTube shows a man standing on a stage, addressing a crowd of protesters.[1] He's wearing a white short-sleeved top – the footage is too grainy to read the circular navy logo over his left breast. His eyes are shielded from the late spring sun with dark glasses. He speaks into the lime green microphone, occasionally looking at his notes. He appears of slight stature, but his passion and his rage make him seem sturdier. This is the celebrated LGBT activist, film historian and author Vito Russo. He's most well-known for his book *The Celluloid Closet*, and for co-founding the Gay and Lesbian Alliance Against Defamation (GLAAD), both focusing on the representation of LGBT people in media and film.

He starts by telling a story about his friend who was questioned by an attendant as to why he was using a discounted New York transit card. When his friend said it was because he had AIDS, the attendant responded with disbelief telling him that he couldn't have the condition – if he did, he would be dying at home, not out and about using public transport. Russo wanted 'to speak out today as a person with AIDS who is not dying'. He goes on to describe how if he is dying, it is from homophobia, racism, bureaucracy, indifference and prejudice, calling out in particular the media, the president of the United States and senator Jesse Helms.* He says powerfully, 'If I'm dying from anything, I'm dying from the fact that not enough rich, white, heterosexual men have gotten AIDS for anybody to give a shit.'[2]

Russo's blistering speech, 'Why We Fight', shows exactly what people living with, and dying from, AIDS were up against in 1988. He died just two years later, on 7 November 1990, one of millions of people who died from AIDS before they had access to effective treatment.[3]

The AIDS epidemic made itself known to the world in 1981. Cases of the rare pneumocystis pneumonia and cancer, Kaposi's sarcoma, started to be reported in clusters of young, previously well gay men in New York, Los Angeles and San Francisco. These were conditions rarely seen in healthy people. Doctors started to see more and more people, mainly gay men, with signs of a failing immune system – severe weight loss, fungal infections, tuberculosis, profuse diarrhoea. Initially called gay-related immune deficiency (GRID), the Centers for Disease Control and Prevention (CDC)

---

*Jesse Helms was an American politician who barred the use of federal funding for HIV/AIDS educational materials that would 'promote or encourage, directly or indirectly, homosexual activities'.

used the term acquired immune deficiency syndrome (AIDS) for the first time in 1982. In 1983 scientists at laboratories in France and the US identified HIV (human immunodeficiency virus) as the cause of AIDS. In 1985, an antibody test was licensed to diagnose people with HIV. This meant that people could see whether they had the virus, but with no effective treatment would know they'd progressively get sicker and die.[4]

The AIDS Coalition to Unleash Power (ACT UP) was formed in the US in 1987 and by then the situation was dire. AIDS had killed over 40,000 people in the US and no drugs were licensed to treat HIV. People with AIDS (as they preferred to call themselves rather than AIDS 'victims' or 'carriers') had realised that they were being forsaken by the people in power who were meant to be protecting them. Famously, President Ronald Reagan did not even mention AIDS publicly until 1985, four years after the epidemic started in the US. At this time, people with AIDS were facing a huge amount of discrimination and hate – being fired from their jobs, losing their careers, being banished from their family and being made homeless. They were people who were already marginalised by society – LGBTQ+ people, people of colour, people who injected drugs. Discussions about them in the media and politics were alarming – conservative political pundit William F. Buckley Jr. had written in the *New York Times* that 'AIDS carriers' should be tattooed;[5] politicians had discussed quarantining people with AIDS, separating them from the rest of society and taking away their human rights.[6] It was in this authoritarian climate that the Silence=Death Collective, a group of six consciousness-raising activists, created their famous poster that was integral to ACT UP's campaigning. It consisted of a pink triangle placed above the words 'SILENCE=DEATH' written in white on a black background. They had taken the downward pointing pink triangle, which Nazis in the 1930s and 40s had sewn onto gay men's uniforms in concentration camps, and turned it so it pointed upwards.

People with AIDS and their allies understood that if they were to survive, they were going to have to save themselves. Silence really equalled death. On 10 March 1987 at the New York Lesbian and Gay

Community Services Center, Larry Kramer* gave an eviscerating speech that prompted the creation of ACT UP. Kramer was a well-known playwright, author and gay activist who had co-founded the community group Gay Men's Health Crisis in response to the emerging epidemic in 1982. He delivered a provocation to the assembled crowd: 'You will be dead in five years. Two thirds of you will die. What are you going to do to save yourselves?' He went on to tell them it would be their fault if they died, they must have a death wish as they have allowed themselves to be killed, by not fighting back.[7]

It worked. Two days later, more than 300 people gathered at the same Lesbian and Gay Community Services Center on West 13th Street, New York, and formed ACT UP. They met every Monday night in a room on the ground floor of the center. Each meeting started with a recital of ACT UP's motto, 'The AIDS Coalition to Unleash Power is a diverse, non-partisan group of individuals, united in anger and committed to direct action to end the AIDS crisis.'

At ACT UP's height it is said that up to 800 people attended meetings, sitting on metal chairs or standing on the green and black chequered linoleum floor. These were people with AIDS, their friends and loved ones, concerned members of the public and activists from other social justice movements. They came together with an urgency and drive to make a difference. They were mostly young, and as daily witnesses to suffering, illness and death, they were desperate. They couldn't turn away from the problem and they didn't have time to waste. This made them more effective as agents of change. People took it in turns to stand up and speak on the microphone with an idea or thought. Other members listened, commented and argued. Footage from documentaries like *United*

---

*Larry Kramer's most famous play, *The Normal Heart*, is a largely autobiographical account about Gay Men's Health Crisis. It's still widely performed around the world. I first saw it in Washington in 2012, when attending the International AIDS Society Conference. This was the first time it had been performed in the US since the government lifted its travel ban for foreign nationals with HIV, two years earlier.

in Anger: A History of ACT UP and *How to Survive a Plague*, show just how electrifying the atmosphere in the room was.[8, 9]

This group did change the world. In just a few years they forced the government and pharmaceutical companies to transform their priorities in medical research. They influenced how drug trials were run; they changed the CDC definition of AIDS to include conditions that affected women, allowing them to access benefits and social support; they made needle exchange legal to reduce transmission of HIV between people using drugs; they started Housing Works to support homeless people with AIDS and their families; they changed the way in which LGBTQ+ people and people with AIDS were viewed – from victims to heroes fighting for their rights; they ended the exclusion of people with AIDS from insurance policies; and they confronted the Catholic Church, who opposed public school condom distributions, needle exchange and abortion.[10] This is such an astonishing list and it continues to directly affect my clinical practice daily, particularly when it comes to treatment and thinking about patients holistically. Why was ACT UP so effective?

The writer Sarah Schulman, who was a member of ACT UP from 1987–92, believes it was due to several approaches: using pre-existing methods of non-violent civil disobedience, affinity groups and an 'Insider–Outsider' strategy. Schulman, together with filmmaker Jim Hubbard, interviewed 188 surviving members of ACT UP between 2002–18. These make up the ACT UP Oral History Project, which aims to ensure that the history of HIV activism is visible and accessible. In her book *Let the Record Show: A Political History of ACT UP New York, 1987–1993*, Schulman writes that 'It was a very human, complex, multifaceted society of activists who succeeded in winning significant victories, against great odds, that changed the world and literally saved lives.'[11]

The methods of non-violent civil disobedience were learnt from pre-existing social movements in the fifties, sixties and seventies such as those supporting LGBTQ+ rights. These included public demonstrations which directly confronted the people in power by those affected. These could be loud and theatrical, like in 1991 when ACT UP members unrolled a giant condom over the roof of Senator

Jesse Helms' house. Or quiet, like the die-ins where people lay still on the ground in public spaces, such as in St Patrick's Cathedral at the Stop the Church Action in 1989. These were designed to shame people in power, and with media outlets projecting the images of these actions to the rest of the world, achieved this aim.

ACT UP used 'affinity groups' to be able to work at speed. This was a concept from civil rights and feminist movements where small groups of people concentrated on one area of activism and worked simultaneously with other groups. It meant that a consensus from the whole ACT UP group was not required for an action to be agreed on, which would have taken time.

By 1996, just thirteen years since HIV was isolated, effective treatment was discovered and HIV no longer carried with it the certainty of premature death.

*

An integral part of my job is to prescribe drugs that treat HIV to people I see in clinic and on the wards. Day to day, I see first hand how they make people feel better and healthier by controlling the virus and letting the body's immune system recover. In 2023, I have the luxury of choosing from a range of more than thirty HIV drugs from six different classes, which work in different ways to stop the virus from replicating. These medicines have fewer side effects and can be given together in a single daily tablet or by injection every two months. This means that I can now tailor therapy to a person's needs and wants. And it works! People living with HIV can live long, healthy lives and have families. Life expectancy is now the same as the general population. We also have the evidence to show that if someone is on effective treatment with an undetectable viral load, they cannot pass HIV on through sex. This, along with the increased availability of HIV testing and the prevention medication PrEP (pre-exposure prophylaxis), means that we have the scientific tools to end HIV as a public health threat.

Without patients and other activists shouting for treatment, this would not be possible. In 1987, just after ACT UP formed, AZT (also known as Zidovudine), the first drug to treat HIV, was approved. In the early 1980s as the number of people with AIDS started to increase, pharmaceutical companies first looked at the existing drugs they already had on their shelves. AZT was a failed nucleoside drug created in the 1950s to treat cancer. It never got to the stage of being tested in humans as it was too toxic. However, in the 1980s it was found in lab tests to stop HIV from reproducing and making more virus, and so was tested in humans. A randomised controlled trial recruited 300 people with AIDS from clinics across the US, and initial results showed that AZT seemed to improve the survival rates of those taking it. In the placebo arm (consisting of those who were not on AZT) nineteen people died within seventeen weeks. In the AZT arm, one person died. The trial was stopped early as it was not deemed ethical to continue and deny half of its participants an apparently effective drug which could lengthen their life.

The company that made AZT was Burroughs, Wellcome & Co., co-founded by Henry Wellcome, who we met in Chapter 4. As soon as AZT started to be considered as a possible treatment for HIV, the company patented the drug, stopping others from making and potentially gaining financially from it. It was approved in March 1987 and by 1989 was the drug making the highest profits globally, costing an individual patient $10,000 a year. It was not without its detractors – AZT was given at such high doses that it had terrible side effects including anaemia, muscle pain, vomiting, fatigue and loss of appetite due to a persistent change in taste. Its efficacy and safety were questioned at the time by some patients and medical professionals, who were later proved right. AZT would be found to cause no improvement in the survival of people with AIDS, as the virus quickly mutated, causing drug resistance. The Concorde trial in 1993 confirmed that AZT did not prevent AIDS or death.[12]

In 1987, however, this wasn't known and AZT was the only drug approved to treat HIV. People with AIDS were agitating for more. Within ACT UP, they were led by Treatment and Data, an affinity group whose focus was on drugs. They wanted to get existing experimental drugs released early; to ensure drugs were available through fairly enrolled trials; and to make sure people with AIDS knew about these trials and how to get on them. And finally, they wanted new drugs to be developed – not only drugs against HIV, but those to treat and prevent opportunistic diseases. These were conditions that took advantage of the weakened immune systems of people with AIDS and killed them.

Each member of Treatment and Data would choose an experimental drug and research it thoroughly, reading the literature and even ringing up the lead scientists running the drug trials to quiz them. They would then present this information back to the group. One of the members, Iris Long, was a retired chemist who taught the others about how clinical trials and drug approvals were carried out. Using freedom of information requests, the group obtained drug trial protocols, which explicitly documented every aspect of how a trial was to be carried out. They used these to publish the AIDS Treatment Registry, which listed trial sites nationally. This explained how people could get into a drug trial and what it entailed, its risks and benefits. This helped people with AIDS make decisions about their care and was also distributed to doctors who could signpost their patients to trial centres.

Treatment and Data had several concerns about existing drug research and approval processes. Firstly, they thought the Food and Drug Administration (FDA) took too long to approve drugs. People dying could not wait the average four to seven years to approval. They also criticised 'gold standard' double-blind randomised controlled trials for being unethical. These trials used placebos, sugar pills with no therapeutic effects designed to look like the experimental drug. Doctors did not know who on the trial were going to get placebos and potentially die and who had a chance of living with the experimental drug. Some of these trials included children with HIV who were often poor, Black or Hispanic. ACT UP members felt that they could not consent to be on the trial in a meaningful way. Trials had strict inclusion criteria, which often excluded women of childbearing age, anyone the investigators judged may be non-adherent (usually people who were poor, injected drugs or people of colour), people with opportunistic infections and people on another trial drug. This meant trials often could not recruit enough participants, leaving experimental drugs unused. ACT UP members felt that this was a waste of drugs that could potentially save people's lives. Not only that, for many people with AIDS, drugs trials were the only route to accessing healthcare, as they could not afford it otherwise.

Using an Insider–Outsider strategy, 'insider' members of the group would meet with prominent governmental figures such as Anthony Fauci,* director of the NIAID (National Institute of Allergy and Infectious Diseases), part of the NIH (National Institutes of Health). Self-taught, the activists were soon recognised for having sound enough scientific knowledge to be invited onto drug trial committees.

In his book *Impure Science: AIDS, Activism and the Politics of Knowledge*, sociologist Stephen Epstein explored how HIV activists changed paradigms about who is viewed as a source of medical knowledge.[13] By teaching themselves the intricacies of virology, immunology and epidemiology, he felt those in the AIDS movement 'have established their credibility as people who might legitimately speak in the language of medical science'. People living with HIV proved that they were alternative sources of expertise about disease – that of lived and learnt experience. This meant they could represent patient perspectives inside government. It's no coincidence that the ACT UP members who were listened to and invited 'inside' were white men, people who are most likely to be seen as credible, and heard.

The rest of ACT UP worked 'outside', carrying out strategic public demonstrations. One of the most effective demonstrations was the Seize Control of the FDA (Food and Drug Administration) action. This forced a change in the definition of 'expanded access', giving people excluded from trials access to experimental medication on compassionate grounds. These were people who didn't fit strict inclusion criteria for drug trials and gave them a chance to potentially

---

* Fauci was Director of the National Institute of Allergy and Infectious Diseases from 1984 to 2022, working on public health crises, including most recently COVID-19, where he was often seen to publicly disagree with the then president, Donald Trump.

get better. This was ACT UP's first national mobilisation and its first major victory. On 11 October 1988, 1,000 people gathered at the FDA buildings in leafy, suburban Maryland, pressurising them to cut the bureaucratic red tape involved in lengthy drug approval processes. People held die-ins or marched with signs painted to look like grave stones with slogans painted on them, such as 'Dead from lack of drugs'. There were protestors in white coats with bloody handprints on them, chanting 'The FDA has blood on its hands and we're seeing red'. A clever media strategy conceived by the journalist members of ACT UP made this national news, contributing to how people with AIDS were viewed – from victims to heroes.

As you may imagine, ACT UP's actions proved popular with pharmaceutical companies who appreciated their drugs being approved faster. By the early 1990s there were newer drugs against HIV and to prevent and treat opportunistic infections. In 1992, some members split from ACT UP to form Treatment Action Group, a non-profit community organisation that paid salaries to its staff. This took the 'insider' strategy further, with members working within pharmaceutical companies and drug committees. Treatment Action Group continued to have a strong impact, speeding up the development of drugs and influencing the research agenda.

The early to mid-nineties was a desperate time for ACT UP as many of the activists campaigning in the eighties had died. But in 1996, the miracle that they had been waiting for was finally discovered – effective HIV therapy. Scientists presented evidence at the Vancouver AIDS Conference that combining three HIV drugs (two nucleosides and the new class of protease inhibitors) seemed to not only suppress the virus, but keep it down. Three drugs were needed to stop the virus mutating and causing drug resistance. The news quickly spread and doctors around the world started to prescribe these drugs to their patients. In 1998, a large study of 1,255 patients in the US showed that death rates had dramatically declined among patients on this combination therapy.[14]

People with AIDS who had survived long enough to access this treatment could start to think about the rest of their lives.

Both ACT UP and Treatment Action Group continue to operate

to this day. ACT UP has 148 chapters around the world, and its activists have instigated change at local and international levels. Schulman wrote that one of the reasons they carried out the ACT UP Oral History Project was to ensure that activists of the future could learn lessons from the past to make them more effective organisers. She says, 'We wanted to show, clearly, what we had witnessed in ACT UP: that people from all walks of life working together can change the world.'

It still takes my breath away to write about these advances. We really have come so far in just forty years. However, 33 million people have died of AIDS and we still do not have a cure or a vaccine. HIV stigma remains depressingly common. Compare this with COVID-19, a disease that has affected everyone, not just the most marginalised in society – a vaccine was licensed within a year. What could have been achieved if political will and investment had been present from the start of the HIV epidemic? I can't help wondering whether I would now be prescribing a cure.

*

HIV/AIDS is a critical reminder of how not everyone's lives are valued to the same degree around the world by those in power. Not everyone got access to life-saving combination therapy immediately. The situation was very different for the world's poor, living in countries in the Global South who had to keep on fighting for years to access drugs which were too expensive for them. The battle for global access to lower-cost HIV medication is told in *Fire in the Blood*, a 2013 documentary by Dylan Mohan Gray.[15] At the start the narrator says, 'If it is true that one death is a tragedy and a million deaths a statistic, this is a story about statistics. The millions of people in poor countries who died needlessly of AIDS while giant pharmaceutical companies blocked access to the low-cost medicine which could have saved their lives.'[16]

During the eighties and nineties, AIDS had a catastrophic impact on people in countries all around the world, especially in sub-Saharan Africa where there were millions of deaths. This did not change with the introduction of combination treatment in

1996, which at $12,000 a year was too expensive for most Africans to be able to afford. By 2001, just 1 in 2,000 Africans with HIV was being treated. It was a health emergency. A turning point was July 2000, when the International AIDS Conference was held in Durban, its first time in Africa where the majority of people with AIDS lived and died. Protestors amassed outside buildings where the latest scientific research was being examined. They roared that the life-saving antiretroviral drugs that were being discussed were out of reach for most people. They forced the world to watch – it could no longer avert its eyes and let more than 20 million Africans die of AIDS.

At this time, countries such as India, Brazil and Thailand were manufacturing their own generic versions of HIV drugs. Generics are medications which contain the same active ingredients as branded drugs but may be made slightly differently or have different additives. They are generally much cheaper. For example, the Indian generics company Cipla, led by Yusuf Hamied, offered to sell combination antiretroviral treatment for $350 a year or $1 a day (compared to $12,000 a year for branded versions) to countries in Africa.[17] He was blocked by lawsuits from international pharmaceutical companies who held the patents to the drugs. The drug companies were worried that patients in the Global North would question why their drugs were costing so much more than those elsewhere, and that this would affect their profits. Shamefully, these companies were backed up by the political might of Western governments such as the United States, which shows how widely ingrained these systematic barriers were. There were also concerns that generic medication would not be of the same quality as branded, but there was little evidence that this was the case.

The rejection of the $1 a day offer for generic drugs made news headlines and caused global public outrage. Eventually drug companies were forced to waive their patents. In 2003, George Bush announced the launch of The President's Emergency Plan for AIDS Relief (PEPFAR) which committed to expanding access to HIV medications. This, along with other funders, went on to provide generic medication to many countries around the world. By 2022, it was reported that PEPFAR had spent $90 billion on HIV/AIDS treatment, prevention, and research.[18]

While I was somewhat aware that access to HIV treatment around the world had been unequal, watching *Fire in the Blood* alerted me to the gross injustices involved. Policymakers in the Global North were opposed to giving HIV treatment to Africans for reasons which were described as racist.[19] I agree with this. For example, in 2001 Andrew Natsios, the head of the United States Agency for International Development, gave a justification to the US Congress for the agency's opposition, which included that Africans 'do not know what watches and clocks are. They do not use western means for telling time. They use the sun. These drugs have to be administered during a certain sequence of time during the day and when you say take it at 10:00, people will say what do you mean by 10:00?'[20]

Let this sink in. This was at a meeting discussing how 80 million people could die of HIV by 2010, of which 70 per cent would be African. Natsios went on to apologise for these remarks.[21] However, opponents of the decision to give Africans treatment suggested that one of the main reasons was fear that they would not take HIV medication properly, driving widespread HIV drug resistance so existing therapies would no longer work. This was seen as a threat to people living in high-income countries in the Global North, who were at the time benefiting from drugs that worked and kept them alive. Unsurprisingly, they were proved wrong. Research in 2007 showed that Africans were better at taking HIV medications than North Americans.[22] In a commentary piece, one of the authors of this research, Amir Attaran, wrote that, 'Dismissing patients in this way leads to a lower standard of medical care', an integral theme of this book.[23]

Collective patient activism has been instrumental in ensuring HIV treatment has become affordable. One of the main groups involved was the South Africa-based Treatment Action Campaign co-founded on 10 December 1998 by Zackie Achmat, an anti-apartheid campaigner, and colleagues. This was intentionally set on World Human Rights Day, fifty years after the adoption of the

Universal Declaration of Human Rights, to clearly demonstrate the group's intent to fight for the human right to health. Treatment Action Campaign concentrated on getting medications to people who could not afford them. Having initially tried and then failed to encourage pharmaceutical companies to be more transparent about drug pricing, Treatment Action Campaign worked with activists abroad to create a global movement to stop profiteering by drug companies.[24] Together, they challenged patents and the Trade-Related Aspects of Intellectual Property Rights (TRIPS) agreement in countries that had high numbers of people with HIV, tuberculosis and malaria – all treatable conditions if medication was available. Importantly, they worked against what former General Secretary of Treatment Action Campaign Vuyiseka Dubula calls 'a denialist government' in South Africa that 'went so far as to publicly refute the crisis in the health system'.[25] President Thabo Mbeki and his health ministry did not believe that HIV caused AIDS, and so advocated for the use of alternative therapies such as garlic over life-saving HIV antiretroviral therapy.[26] To combat this policy, Treatment Action Campaign mobilised communities. In 2002–3 they went door to door to educate people about the science behind HIV and treatment, and their right to health. By 2004, the government changed direction and antiretroviral HIV therapy became its preferred treatment. Scandalously, it's been estimated that 330,000 people died prematurely and 35,000 babies were born with HIV because they couldn't access antiretroviral therapy.[27]

In her TEDx Talk, Vuyiseka Dubula describes her work in Treatment Action Campaign as its general secretary.[28] She emphasises the importance of solidarity, saying 'It is your business. When there is an injustice, it is your business' and how when TAC went door to door, they spread hope as well as education. Treatment Action Campaign continues to operate in South Africa and has over 8,000 members and a network of 182 branches.

It is estimated that ten million people in the Global South died of AIDS, because they were denied access to affordable medication by pharmaceutical companies and governments in the West. Sadly, access to HIV treatment and prevention around the world remains inequitable. A report by UNAIDS declared that by June 2020, 38 million people were living with HIV globally, of which 26 million (two-thirds) had access to treatment. Just under half of children aged 0–14 years living with HIV globally do not have access to life-saving HIV therapy.[29] In 2022, 1.3 million were newly diagnosed and 630,000 people died of HIV-related conditions.[30] Inequalities are seen between countries and within countries, with the poorest and most marginalised people still bearing the brunt of HIV. UNAIDS has called for an end to these inequalities with a strategic plan focusing on key populations. This requires an increase in investment by governments and funders of $8.5 billion. If we really want to end HIV as a public health threat and save lives, political will and solidarity across continents is needed. People living with HIV and their allies still need to speak up and demand that they are heard – not just by doctors and researchers, but by governments and funders. The need for activism has not finished, we must keep going until everyone has the healthcare that they are entitled to.

*

Who a disease predominantly affects influences how much patients are listened to and how much they are silenced, as individuals and as groups. This in turn influences how much resource is put into addressing the disease, the research done and how much knowledge we have about it. To understand this better, imagine if HIV had only affected people in the Global South. Would we have had such fast scientific progress? Would we have such effective HIV treatment now?

For sociologist Stephen Epstein, writing in 1998, it mattered that AIDS affected white middle-class gay men in the US and Europe, as they had 'a degree of political clout and fundraising capacity unusual for an oppressed group'. He explained that this was because within gay communities were many professionals who worked in science, education and the arts, which gave them a great deal of 'cultural capital'.[31] The members of ACT UP who were invited 'inside' to speak to government and pharmaceutical companies were white middle-class gay men. From the diverse activist group, they were most likely to be seen as credible sources of knowledge. As we know from the concept of epistemic injustice, white middle-class men are one of the groups most likely to be heard, seen as being sincere and taken seriously. So, if HIV/AIDS had just affected Black and brown people in the world's poorest countries, they would not have had this social capital. By the enduring inequity they face in accessing drugs, we know that their lives continue to be less valued by people with power in the Global North.

If we compare HIV to another global disease, tuberculosis (TB), we can see this more clearly. TB has been around for a very long time, first documented in India and China more than 2,000 years ago. Until the twentieth century, when antibiotics were discovered, TB was often fatal. John Keats, the English poet, died from TB at the age of twenty-five. TB can affect anyone, but as it is airborne (spread through air transmission), it is more likely to affect the poor who live in crowded and often unsanitary conditions. Once treatment was discovered, those that could afford the lengthy course of antibiotics were cured. Now TB remains most likely to be seen in countries in the Global South and among impoverished and socially marginalised communities in the Global North. The area of London where I work has a high burden of TB compared to the rest of the UK. TB still kills, causing 1.6 million deaths a year around the world. It was announced as a global emergency by the World Health Organization in 1993, but progress on reducing it globally has been slow compared to other infections.[32] As it is an airborne infection, fear of transmission has meant that it remains stigmatised and that people with TB have been subject to discriminatory practices and social exclusion such as forced quarantine – violations of their human rights.

In 2023 I was invited by visiting professor Madhukar Pai to attend his lecture at the London School of Hygiene and Tropical Medicine. Pai is passionate about health equity and, in particular, improving TB care. In his talk, he emphasised how far we still had to go with TB, in that we still don't have adequate diagnostic tests; the only vaccine we have started being used in 1921 and offers little protection; and that access to the newer and shorter antibiotic treatment regimens are restricted. I was struck by his comparisons with HIV, where he felt that the speed of scientific progress was much faster. He theorised that patient voices had been less heard in TB than HIV over the years and perhaps this was the reason.

This was my first time inside the London School of Hygiene and Tropical Medicine, an organisation that has been an integral part of global health, and which has been recently examining its role in colonialism.[33] As I sat in the lecture hall feeling the weight of its history, it became evident to me that as TB mainly affected Black and brown people who make up the world's poor, this was why their voices were not being heard. This was racism.

In Pai's lecture, I learnt how patient voice was starting to be more incorporated in TB research and service development. Grassroots activist networks such as the Stop TB Partnership, Treatment Action Group, TB Proof, Global Coalition of Tuberculosis Activists and KNCV Tuberculosis Foundation are working to combat stigma and agitate for a more human rights-based approach to TB care.[34]

Nandita Venkatesan is a survivor of two life-threatening bouts of the disease, requiring six operations and resulting in being bed-bound for two years and losing her hearing. Now a prominent TB activist and journalist, she is a vocal advocate for better care. She gave a powerful speech at the UN General Assembly's first High-Level Meeting on Tuberculosis in 2018, where she said, 'Survivors bring to the table first-hand experience of ground realities, empathy, and a burning desire to shake the status quo. Use them, not think for us, without us.'[35]

Patient voices are essential for us to agitate for change and I am hopeful that such voices will be followed by improvements in tuberculosis care and treatment around the world. Perhaps this would have happened more quickly had TB mainly affected people in the Global North.

*

Patient activism has been a driving force for change in the UK, too. My work has been infinitely enriched by my colleagues with lived experience of HIV – those working in and leading charities, patient activists and peer support workers. They have transformed my approach to medicine and I'm certain that this book would not exist without what they've taught me over the years. I'm humbled by their strength and knowledge and I have actively sought out opportunities to work with them in my voluntary roles. Activists in the UK during the HIV/AIDS epidemic also changed medicine, their voices coming together to be heard.

The AIDS epidemic emerged in the UK at the start of the 1980s, initially being seen in the gay community. One of the first-known people who died of AIDS was Terry Higgins, a Welshman who worked at the Houses of Parliament, and as a DJ and barman in London. He collapsed at the LGBTQ+ nightclub Heaven and died from AIDS-related conditions on 4 July 1982. He was thirty-seven years old.[36] Like in the US, while the government took its time to address HIV/AIDS as serious issue, patients and the communities they belonged to in the UK had to mobilise to save themselves. Terry's partner Rupert Whitaker and friend Martyn Butler founded the Terrence Higgins Trust in his memory, the first charity created in response to the epidemic, which remains the largest in the UK to this day. Their aim was initially to raise money for research into what at that point was a mystery disease. They soon realised there was so much more to do with raising awareness and supporting people. By naming the charity after Terry, they also wanted to humanise people with AIDS. Higgins' life has since been commemorated in many ways, including in the award-winning 2022 BBC podcast *A Positive Life: HIV from Terrence Higgins to Today*, which I contributed to.[37] The producers interviewed friends from throughout his life, who shared personal details with us. It was illuminating to hear more about him. One common theme was his love for dancing, and his distinctive style, described as 'a human slinky' and 'wiggle-legs'.

Existing charities were also integral to the AIDS response. The London Lesbian and Gay Switchboard had launched in 1974 as a resource for the LGBTQ+ community in London. It became the main source of advice and solace for people in the 1980s who were affected by AIDS. There were so many enquiries that staff compiled a directory so that the volunteers could give accurate information to callers. This was the National AIDS Manual, then a huge ring binder full of papers, which exists to this day as aidsmap, an online information charity, which I often signpost my patients to and contribute to, by reviewing their materials and taking part in educational webinars.[38]

Patients and charities started to collaborate with healthcare professionals. On 21 May 1983 the London Lesbian and Gay Switchboard, along with the Gay Medical Association, hosted the first conference addressing AIDS, at Conway Hall in central London. They invited activists and doctors from the UK and US to present. Looking at the agenda, I'm reminded of how recent this history is. One of the speakers was my now-retired colleague Dr Tom McManus.

As cases of HIV increased, so did fear and discrimination of the groups most affected. In particular, homophobia was rife and openly declared in the media and by politicians. Headlines such as 'Britain Threatened by Gay Virus Plague' in the *Mail on Sunday* were not uncommon.[39] As seen around the world, UK activists were making their case known, loudly and proudly. Like the New York chapter, the London branch of ACT UP had their own giant condom moment. In 1989 activists unfurled a 55m-long cellophane sheath over Nelson's Column in Trafalgar Square. Mass die-ins were held to protest the misrepresentation of people with AIDS and the LGBTQ+ community by the media.[40]

Patient activists also changed the way medical care is delivered. In April 1987 Princess Diana officially opened Broderip Ward at the Middlesex Hospital, the first in the UK dedicated to treating people with AIDS. The princess was photographed by the world's media talking with patients and holding their hands, showing clearly that HIV could not be passed on through touch, a huge step to reducing stigma. Broderip Ward was groundbreaking, changing traditional models of nursing and medical care. Many people with AIDS had faced prejudice from healthcare workers on hospital wards, feeling they were being blamed for being ill. At the start of the epidemic, nurses and doctors wore excessive personal protective equipment for fear of infection; patients were kept in side rooms on their own, with their meals being left outside the door; partners and friends were not allowed to visit as deemed not family.

In the UK, by 1987, as scientific knowledge about HIV transmission had progressed, these practices had changed, and staff describe the close relationships they developed with patients. On Broderip Ward, partners could stay overnight with their loved ones – mattresses were provided, although staff tell of how they pretended not to know that the couples shared hospital beds. The ward had plenty of visitors with parties held by drag artists and other entertainers. Without effective treatment, the aim was to ensure people made the most of the lives they had left. This put patients at the centre of treatment. In the podcast series *We Were Always Here*, HIV activist Marc Thompson talks to Jane Bruton, who was a nurse on Broderip Ward.[41] With much laughter, she tells a memorable story of a patient whose last wish was to do a bungee jump before he died. Amazingly, the ward staff arranged for this to happen and when he did, his false teeth fell out, a moment which was apparently captured on camera!

Photographer Gideon Mendel memorialised the ward in images in 1993, which have since been exhibited.[42] These are achingly moving and intimate, conveying more than any words can – a man and his partner kissing on a bed, a nurse having a free shiatsu massage for stress relief, patients being visited by family and friends. Seeing these photos, I think about how different my ward rounds are now. We no longer have a ward dedicated to people with HIV – due to antiretroviral therapy, thankfully there aren't enough patients to fill a ward. Even in my fifteen years in the speciality, the numbers of patients we look after has decreased dramatically. But as a multidisciplinary team we are still dedicated to treating our patients with dignity and care. We still advocate for them and challenge HIV stigma whenever we come across it. Despite so much medical progress, people living with HIV continue to report discrimination from healthcare workers and the wider public, something that should never happen. I see the effects of this stigma from patients who are sick because they have avoided healthcare services due to prior experiences. It's frustrating as a HIV doctor to see this still happen, and I don't think that it's just the responsibility of people living with HIV to address this – it's all of ours. This is an important lesson that I think is relevant for healthcare professionals working in other disease areas. I feel passionately that part of our role involves advocating for our patients in a broader sense as well as treating individuals.

Simon Collins and Winnie Ssanyu Sseruma have worked in the HIV sector for several decades, first meeting at the AIDS Treatment Project in the late 1990s. Simon told me that the aim of this group was 'that people living with HIV should be able to make their own decisions about treatment, not just have these made for us'. They ran a treatment information phone line so people could discuss the new medications that were being introduced at that time. AIDS Treatment Project was volunteer-based and mostly run by people living with HIV, which made it different to most national HIV charities. As they had direct experience of HIV and related infections, and were taking the medications themselves, this gave them a more informed perspective when talking to callers. Collins had been too ill to attend the first meeting, but antiretroviral therapy had so dramatically changed his health that within a month, he was able to volunteer. 'Because I knew the new meds worked, I wanted to become actively involved.'[43]

This was similar to Ssanyu Sseruma, who had experienced the 'Lazarus effect' that was starting to be talked about – that astonishing feeling of coming back from the dead after starting therapy. Her route to the AIDS Treatment Project was via Body and Soul, a charity run by women for families affected by HIV. Body and Soul put women first, providing transport costs, a hot meal and childcare, massages and toiletries. This gave women time to focus on themselves. Ssanyu Sseruma met dozens of other African women there and was persuaded to start treatment having heard their stories. She tells me, 'It was mind-blowing. They gave me the hope to want to live.' She started to attend AIDS Treatment Project meetings, learning about her body, what the virus did to it and how treatment worked. She says, 'Understanding the medical science on how HIV treatments work not only helped me to become an expert patient in my health, but also enabled me to empower others to improve their treatment literacy. Treatment literacy opened up a whole new world for me, a skill that I continue to build on and adapt to other health conditions.'

In 2000, Collins went on to co-found the charity HIV i-Base with colleagues from the AIDS Treatment Project.[44] This is a treatment activist group that publishes technical and non-technical publications for health professionals and people living with HIV, in different formats and languages. It still runs a phone line and is now also contactable by email, and online, answering thousands of questions each year from individuals all around the world. HIV i-Base set up the UK Community Advisory Board (UK-CAB) in 2002. This is a network of HIV advocates, including people living with HIV which now has over 700 members. It is run by an elected steering group and it ensures that patient voices are always included in national treatment guidelines as well as other HIV policy areas.

Over the years, Collins, with the UK-CAB, has been developing increased community involvement in research and treatment guidelines. He is a community advisor for many HIV studies. At conferences, Collins is among a group of HIV advocates who ask some of the most pertinent and detailed questions of scientists. This knowledge of HIV treatment and research is formidable and something I and my colleagues aspire to.

Ssanyu Sseruma went on to work for HIV i-Base with Collins, teaching the treatment literacy programme and working on the phone line. This was the start of many leadership roles in HIV organisations in the UK and abroad, including chairing the African Health Policy Network, working for Christian Aid, UK and the Stephen Lewis Foundation, Canada. Ssanyu Sseruma is also one of the five Black African female editors of *Our Stories Told By Us*, a book that highlights the contribution that African communities have made in the UK's HIV response.[45] Along with Rebecca Mbewe, Angelina Namiba, Charity Nyirenda and Memory Sachikonye, she writes in the introduction, 'In this important period of reflection on over 40 years of the UK's HIV response, we felt it was critical to tell these stories. Above all else, it was pivotal for Africans living with HIV to lead this project and to tell our own stories in our own words. If not now, then when? If not us, then who?' This is powerful, and this book brings to the fore voices which are seldom heard, in their own words. At their book launch, the editors were keen to point out that African women living with HIV had never been 'passive or voiceless victims', they had been unheard, ignored or had their resilience dismissed.

As in other areas of medicine, women have been historically silenced in HIV/AIDS, showing how even within marginalised groups there are those that are more marginalised. As the epidemic progressed in the UK, women started to be diagnosed. There were initially few, but by 1992 this was changing, with 12 per cent of HIV cases in the UK being women.[46] HIV was not regarded as a 'women's disease' and at the beginning, some healthcare workers did not even know that women could get HIV. Once diagnosed many women reported that without effective treatment, they were told there was nothing that could be done for them. They were just advised not to have children – viewing them as vectors of disease rather than humans in their own right, requiring care and support. Charities at the time did have some services for women but were mainly designed for the needs of gay men.[47] It was in this void that Positively Women was formed in London in 1987.[48] It was founded by women who had injected drugs and they used their experience of peer support in recovery programmes and replicated these at Positively Women as a tool for empowerment. This charity continues as Positively UK and has been at the forefront of establishing peer support networks around the UK.[49, 50]

Despite now making up the majority of people living with HIV globally, women are still often left out of mainstream narratives about HIV. This was particularly evident in Channel 4's 2021 series about the start of the AIDS epidemic in London, *It's a Sin*, where there were no HIV-positive female characters.[51] In recent years, campaigns to counter their omission from research and policy have been launched. With names like 'Invisible No Longer' and 'We Are Still Here', it's apparent that despite the progress made, there is still much to do to achieve gender equality in the research and treatment of HIV.[52, 53] This includes for transgender and non-binary people who are disproportionally affected by HIV due to structural and social inequalities, which put them at higher risk of acquiring the virus, as well as discrimination in healthcare settings.[54]

It is now standard practice to involve people living with HIV in national and international research and treatment guideline groups. In 2017 the British HIV Association (BHIVA), which represents UK healthcare professionals, went one step further by appointing Jo Josh, a writer living with HIV and a strategic communications consultant for more than thirty years, to manage its relationship with media, the health system and HIV organisations. She says, 'As an HIV activist I'm very aware that sharing accurate information helps to reduce stigma. As I literally have skin in the game, it's great to use the opportunities offered as Communications Officer for BHIVA.' Josh told me how the role 'has arguably enabled me to use my insight and experience to increase the depth and scope of mainstream media coverage, as well as to ensure everyone can understand treatment guidance'. I worked closely with Josh during the COVID-19 pandemic as I chaired BHIVA's external relations team. Recognising the need for accurate information at speed, we helped create almost weekly updates for medical professionals, plus plain language versions for people living with HIV.

HIV activists have taught and continue to teach the world to be less stigmatising and disempowering, and in the process, they have changed language and terminology around the disease. A recent example is the People First Charter, formed in 2021, which is campaigning for terminology that puts the individual before their condition, such as changing 'injecting drug user' to 'person who injects drugs'; language that is less victim blaming – 'failing patients' to 'people on failing therapy' – and more empowering – changing 'compliant' to 'taking medication as recommended'.[55] This may seem like a minor issue to some healthcare professionals and researchers, but we know from listening to patients that it is an important shift to reframe how they feel about themselves – people are so much more than the disease they have. These are small changes that are easy to make and can have a huge impact.

*

People living with HIV changed the paradigm of what a patient could do. While I have focused on HIV as it is my specialism, there are other examples in the world that demonstrate the power and force of patient voice and activism, such as myalgic encephalo-myelitis/chronic fatigue syndrome (ME/CFS). I have not had the space to include all of them here. HIV activists showed themselves to be a source of alternative medical knowledge to the medical profession, and by doing so, highlighted the importance of lived experience. They have demonstrated how patients must be involved in every aspect of medicine, research and policy as the well-used phrase 'Nothing about us, without us' advocates. We can also see this activism with emerging conditions like long Covid, where people report being dismissed by doctors. HIV activists have provided hope that the management of these conditions can improve. What lessons can be learnt from these HIV/AIDS activists for other patient activists?

Firstly, the value of peer support as a means of empowerment and building community. This is well-established not only in HIV, but in areas such as mental health. Recently, it has been introduced in diabetes care. Positively UK (previously Positively Women) have led the way with peer support in Britain, including writing national standards which cover training and supervision for peer support workers. The authors of the national standards say, 'At the roots of peer support there is a hope and a belief that through sharing and support we can transform our lives and the lives of our communities for the better.'[56]

Secondly, treatment literacy: learning about the scientific aspects of the disease, available treatments and current research. This earns patients credibility and respect from the medical profession, which means they are more likely to be heard and viewed as experts in their own condition.

Thirdly, leadership: both Winnie Ssanyu Sseruma and Simon

Collins talked about how health charities and organisations must include more people with lived experience of the condition and they should be in leadership, driving direction. This is not always the case – I spoke to Rebecca Tayler Edwards (who we met in Chapter 1) about this. She works at a disability organisation and said, 'In spaces that consider disability, disability charities and committees that are run by able-bodied people are more widely recognised, funded and endorsed by our society. This is widely accepted, and when our voices are considered, space is rarely made for our intersectional testimonies.' She went on, 'So, my work as a disabled person, developing organisations run by, and for, disabled people, acts to resist the norm. It lobbies for the recognition that we are experts in society and holds policymakers, academic institutions and funders to account for that recognition through tangible action.'

Fourthly, solidarity: different groups recognising their similarities and working with each other. Collins spoke of how HIV i-Base in the UK has worked with Treatment Access Campaign in South Africa to support treatment literacy. This included a project called 'Modern ART for South Africa' that produced a variety of resources to keep rural South Africans informed of newer HIV treatments, which are potentially life-changing.[57, 58] Collins said the experience HIV i-Base had 'from the privilege of being involved, and from working with TAC activists' was also life-changing.

Finally, sharing learning: Ssanyu Sseruma is passionate about this, emphasising that contrary to tradition, learning must flow from the Global South to the North and from younger generations to older. She is setting up a new organisation training health champions in Black communities to help people advocate for themselves and as a group, saying, 'Being able to advocate for myself is empowering. I need to share that.'

*

The *Oxford English Dictionary* describes a patient as being:

noun
A person receiving or registered to receive medical treatment.

It also describes the word 'patient' as:

adjective
Able to accept or tolerate delays, problems, or suffering
without becoming annoyed or anxious.

The word originates from Latin *patient-* 'suffering', from the
verb *pati* (to suffer).[59]

These definitions suggest that patients are passive or even sub-
ordinate, but as we've seen, this is not true. Patients have spoken
up throughout history, but this may not have been documented. I
spoke to historian Anne Hanley about this. She told me about how
many records are from institutions and as such, written by doctors.
Patients from marginalised groups such as the poor, women and the
illiterate either didn't leave written material, or it wasn't valued and
was destroyed. This highlights just how long the history of marginalised peoples' voices being erased is. With Jessica Meyer, Hanley
co-edited a book of essays, *Patient Voices in Britain, 1840–1948*.[60] The
essays are a fascinating read, showing how patients have used their
agency over the years. These included examples of co-producing
healthcare services, developing their own understandings of medicine guided by shared lived experiences and creating vernacular
medical practices (such as herbal medicine or spiritual healing).
This is patients learning about how to heal themselves, giving them a
power outside of the biomedical healthcare system. This collection of
essays is a valuable reminder for health policymakers that healthcare
is also undertaken by those outside of the professional sector.

Patient organisations for many difference conditions have had
a huge impact on healthcare and research around the world. The
Patients Association is an independent charity which campaigns for
better health and social care for patients in the UK. It has a helpline
to support people with their concerns about their care and also
speaks with the government and policymakers to 'ensure the patient
voice is heard and acted upon'.[61] The International Alliance of
Patients' Organizations and World Patients Alliance are international

umbrella organisations, which work with global health institutions like the World Health Organization to perform the same role at a larger scale.[62, 63] Sociologists Peter Wehling and Willy Viehöver have written about how patient activists have challenged paternalistic models of medicine to 'publicly reshape the idea of active patients as knowledgeable subjects or even powerful partners'.[64] In David Gilbert's *The Patient Revolution*, patient leaders emphasise that many of the skills that patients have through coping with their illness and navigating healthcare, such as resilience, passion and humanity are those that are seen as being 'good leadership skills'. They are inherently problem-solvers, able to identify gaps in and between healthcare services, and bring a new perspective to resolving them. In short, they ensure that decisions made about the healthcare service are better quality.[65]

One critique of patient organisations is that they can become influenced by pharmaceutical companies to advocate for the approval of medications that may not always be recommended by doctors. However, I think this is a more general problem for the medical profession and researchers, as well as patient groups. We need strict regulation to ensure that there is transparency about who funds research, organisations and campaigns, and that any conflicts of interest are always declared.

Throughout history, patients have fought back against systems of unaccountable power that have tried to silence them and changed the way we produce scientific knowledge and practice medicine. To improve healthcare, we need to hear patients. This requires systematic ways of supporting patients to speak up and an infrastructure for this. If we truly want a more equal healthcare system, then we need to listen more ethically to patients, particularly the most marginalised.

Summary: Lessons from patients on how to be heard in healthcare

- Create community – link up with other people affected by the condition to share experiences and empower others.
- Lobby for the training and use of peer support workers. They have an expertise that healthcare professionals cannot provide and can help bring community to people who are isolated with their illness.
- Develop treatment literacy at an individual and group level. This helps build credibility to interact on an equal footing with the medical and scientific sectors.
- Collaborate with other groups and across sectors.
- Solidarity – where different groups recognise their similarities and work with each other.
- Sharing learning – disseminate the successes and pitfalls so other groups can learn from them.
- Leadership – while it is not essential for leaders of organisations to have lived experience, it can be very powerful when they do.

7

Justice

How to Listen Ethically

Take this pen, my paper, these words,
But I promise you no applause.
For applause implies the work has ended.

From The Unsung, *a poem by Hanan Issa, National Poet of Wales, to mark the 75th birthday of the National Health Service in 2023*[1]

For one minute at 8 p.m. every Thursday evening during the first COVID-19 lockdown, the streets of Britain were filled with noise. People opened their windows or stood in their gardens to clap and cheer, banging pots and pans to show their appreciation for frontline health and social care workers. This was Clap for Carers, an initiative originating in the Netherlands and brought to the UK by a Dutch woman, Annemarie Plas, who lived in London. It went on to include all key workers. It's thought that millions of people took part in this communal activity, approximately 69 per cent of the British population.

Before the first clap on 26 March 2020, I didn't know what to expect. As a sexual health doctor, I joked how 'the clap' had always held very different connotations for me – being used as a collo-quial term for gonorrhoea. Like many of my colleagues, I was also apprehensive and a bit cynical about it. I didn't want applause and I didn't want to be treated as a hero. I wanted personal protective equipment, safe working conditions and adequate remuneration for key workers. I wondered whether members of the public would even take part. But as I sat on the sofa at 8 p.m., recovering from yet another busy and bewildering day at work, I heard a wave of noise rapidly increasing in volume on my street. I looked out of the window to see dozens of my neighbours clapping to show their gratitude. It unexpectedly moved me, an emotion that I discovered was shared by many frontline workers. For two months this continued on a weekly basis, a regular little boost during this strange period of life.

While Clap for Carers helped to keep morale up, many people felt that it was an insufficient substitute for more substantial support such as longer-term investment in health and social care.[2] There was also considerable fear that the clap may at some point in the future turn into a slap. As the pandemic dragged on and healthcare services became increasingly stretched, many anticipated that people would start to feel frustrated, taking their anger out on frontline staff. We would no longer be seen as 'Covid heroes' (a term that many, including me, rejected). We also knew that once the pandemic had subsided, we would need to catch up with all the elective work that had been delayed – operations, clinic appointments, treatments. There would be no rest for us. And more than four years on from the start of the pandemic, we can see that many of these fears have materialised, with hostile media rhetoric about 'lazy, greedy doctors' and public satisfaction with the NHS falling to its lowest in forty years.[3, 4] The effect of this on the healthcare workforce has meant many staff have left, leading to high levels of job vacancies, increased numbers of staff on sick leave and multiple professional groups are striking.[5]

By spring 2021, in the aftermath of a particularly devastating wave of COVID-19, I decided that I needed to plan a sabbatical. I was physically and mentally drained. With the support of my colleagues and family, I applied for a full-time masters in social epidemiology. I reasoned that this would provide me with the opportunity to learn new skills useful for future research in health inequalities, as well as the break I needed from clinical practice, my first in almost twenty years. I left work at the end of September and by Christmas

I had come to understand that the old adage 'a change is as good as rest' was not true for me. I was enjoying the masters, which was challenging my brain in new ways, but it was more work than I had expected. I was still exhausted, but it didn't feel like this was just due to studying. Why was I feeling like this?

Like the rest of the world, I had found living through the COVID-19 pandemic hard. As a healthcare worker, I saw its shattering effects first hand, but I don't think that I had it harder than other NHS staff. Yes, there were terrible days such as when I came in to find three of my HIV patients on the wards had died of COVID-19 overnight; the online funerals for colleagues we watched at work; the constant changes in routine that were isolating and unsettling. But I was also very lucky to have no one close to me in my personal life who died or became very ill. Although I got COVID-19, it wasn't severe and I didn't get long-lasting effects. I also didn't suffer any financial hardship and I had support from family and friends.

I realised that there was another reason for my exhaustion. I had taken on a whole other strand of work that I continued to do after starting the masters, which I had discounted. This was the work of talking and teaching about racism and health. The COVID-19 pandemic brought to the fore deep-rooted health inequities, particularly faced by racially minoritised groups. This was augmented by the death of George Floyd and the resurgence of the Black Lives Matter movement in summer 2020. I had been teaching and researching racial health inequities before COVID-19, but this felt increasingly urgent to me as I realised that people (including well-respected scientists) did not understand that racism was the root cause, not genetic or biological differences. We needed to change the conditions in which people worked and lived to reduce their exposure to COVID-19, not blame them for having defective bodies.[6]

During 2020 and 2021, I wrote, taught, podcasted, tweeted and researched racism and health inequities. In 2021 alone, I did forty talks on the topic. With increasing use of Zoom and Microsoft Teams, it suddenly became easier to talk to audiences in faraway places. Instead of getting on a train and taking a whole day out to deliver a session at a national conference or departmental teaching, I just had to log in from my living room. This was a welcome distraction from day-to-day work in the hospital and gave me a wider sense of purpose. It was a subject I was passionate about, one I had expertise in, and one that people wanted to hear about. I remain very grateful for the opportunities that came my way, and it had the effect of raising my professional profile nationally and internationally. I often received emails after the sessions thanking me for teaching and then recommendations to speak elsewhere.

But this was work in addition to my day job, and it wasn't always easy. It involved sharing knowledge with different audiences (healthcare workers and students, researchers, policymakers, patient communities and the general public) in a format that they would understand, anticipating their reactions and responding. The information I was presenting was uncomfortable and could be confronting for some. This often led to difficult questions or silence. Some of the more negative responses I got included,

- 'We are already doing well at this compared with other medical specialities, surely we should just celebrate this?'
- 'This is very depressing. Can you tell us about what we are doing well so we don't feel so bad?'
- 'What does this have to do with us?'
- 'What we are talking about here is not as serious and important as other parts of medicine we are meant to know about.'
- 'I don't believe the evidence you are presenting to us.'
- 'This is too big an issue for us to deal with.'
- 'We weren't taught this in medical school, so it can't be right.'
- 'Science is always objective, so I can't understand why you are saying that some research is biased.'

As most of the sessions were delivered online, instead of the usual debrief and small talk with the people who invited me to speak, I logged off finding myself alone in my living room, wondering if it had gone OK. I often felt cold and shivered for several minutes afterwards, a visceral reaction to the emotions of giving the session. Notably, I didn't have this bodily response when I taught about the treatment of HIV or other clinical topics, which elicited less controversy.

In her piece, 'Feeling Depleted?', feminist philosopher Sara Ahmed talks about how 'Diversity work is emotional work because in part it is work that has to be repeated, again and again. You encounter a brick wall.'[7] This helped me understand that I was doing diversity work, which is why it was more exhausting than other types of teaching that I carry out. The effort of being heard, of trying to make people understand the information and getting pushback from audiences, was also draining. In addition, this work was unpaid and done in my own time, in the evenings and on weekends. No wonder I was tired. I had effectively taken on another job. This kind of unacknowledged work (unacknowledged even by myself), as I grew to find out, is common and often seen as a tax on people from marginalised groups.

Throughout this book, I have conveyed the urgent need to listen better in all levels of medicine and health research because being heard is the first step towards being taken seriously as a patient, a colleague, a researcher and a source of knowledge. It confirms our humanity and gives us dignity. However, not all listening is done well, and sometimes speaking up can be harmful for the speaker and even exploitative. Often, we are silenced because to speak is to face intolerance, disrespect or ignorance. We are silenced because so many don't want to hear what we have to say. Listening and being open to other experiences requires discomfort and what we hear can trigger strong reactions in us, but if we don't give spaces to different voices then we will never learn new ways forward. There is a balance that we need to find here, and this is something I have been contemplating for years. How do we listen in a more ethical way?

*

Michael sits on the stage feeling nervous. The overhead lights are beating down on him and he can feel himself start to sweat. He's at his first medical conference, having been asked to take part in a panel discussion on how to improve care for people admitted to hospital with sickle cell crises. The Chair quietens the audience and introduces the members of the expert panel – a senior doctor, a specialist nurse, a policymaker, an eminent researcher and Michael, who's there to give a patient perspective. The rest of the panel smile at him as he's introduced, which makes him feel more comfortable. He arranges his notes and reminds himself why he's there – to tell the medical audience that they need to improve how they treat patients. He is proud to have been invited to speak, and excited to know that doctors would be listening to *him*. Each panel member speaks for seven minutes on the topic and finally it's his turn.

As Michael talks about his recent admission to hospital with a sickle cell crisis, he feels his nerves start to settle as passion takes over. He covers how he felt dismissed by the medical team, how they made him feel like a nuisance to be dealt with, rather than helped. His voice cracks as he tells the auditorium of how scared he felt, worried that he could die from neglect. The audience is silent, people hanging onto his every word. He goes on to suggest what could have been done to make his experience better. As he stops speaking, there is applause. He can see he has moved people. In the Q&A session, no one asks him a question, but several people thank him for speaking, telling him that he is 'brave' and 'an inspiration' for speaking up. The discussion centres on the urgency of the current situation and how there is much that needs to be done to educate healthcare workers on sickle cell disease.

Then the session is over. The Chair thanks Michael and he exchanges some words with the other panel members who reiterate his courage in relating his experience. They say they'll be in touch with him to discuss projects they are working on, so they can collaborate. He is quietly thrilled by this – perhaps things will change, and he can be a part of this!

Michael heads to the busy lunch hall where he finds himself eating alone among tables of medics and researchers, animatedly networking. He leaves earlier than he'd planned to. On the train home, he starts to feel a bit flat, the surge in adrenaline having dissipated. Some of the more distressing parts of his last few hospital admissions come into his mind. To distract himself from these thoughts, he calls his childhood friend Kaya, who has sickle cell disease and has also spoken in public about her experiences. She asks him how it went and he tells her it had been a good experience – he'd felt important on the panel and people listened to him, but he was now tired and on his way home.

Kaya asks, 'And how much did they pay you for the panel?'

He thinks for a second before replying, 'Well . . . they paid for my train journey and gave me free registration to the whole day. I was planning to go to some other sessions, but then felt too tired to. I've got some marking to finish tonight and a really full day at school tomorrow.'

She exclaims, 'But they didn't pay you an honorarium? That's very strange. They normally offer one straight up when they invite me. I won't speak unless I get at least £150.'

He is surprised, stating that no one had mentioned monetary payment to him. Kaya tells him that it is likely the other members of the panel had been paid, so he should have been too. He feels aggrieved and promises her that if there is a next time, he will ask for a fee.

Six months later, he has mostly forgotten about the conference, and no one from the session has contacted him to involve him in the work they have been doing.

One year later, Michael has another sickle cell crisis severe enough to require hospital admission. His experience of being dismissed and disbelieved is similar, and he is again denied adequate pain relief and an early referral to the specialist haematology team. He re-members the conference then, the good intentions stated, but realises nothing has changed despite his contribution.

Michael had been asked to talk about his lived experience as a patient who has had a lifetime of hospital admissions for sickle cell crises. The request was well-intentioned; the conference organisers understood that patient voice was important and wanted to include it. However, there were several things that could have been done to make Michael feel that it had been worth his time to participate. Firstly, while they invited him due to his patient expertise, they did not value it sufficiently. They did not pay him a speaker's fee like they did for the other panel members. This was despite Michael needing to take a day off work to attend the conference. Travel costs and free registration were not sufficient. Secondly, they did not recognise the emotional labour that Michael was providing. This was different to the work asked of other panel members, who were speaking as part of their day jobs. Michael was being asked to recount difficult experiences, to essentially relive his trauma again for the benefit of the medical audience. To do this, he should have been offered some additional support, starting from the acknowledgement that this work is potentially distressing, to follow up afterwards to check that he was OK. Thirdly, despite their interest in his opinion and their expressions of wanting to work with him, he was not contacted after the event to collaborate. And to his knowledge, despite talk of action, he could not see any changes in sickle cell disease policy or guidance. The next time he was admitted with a sickle cell crisis, he suffered the same negative attitudes and neglect from healthcare staff in hospital. It made him feel that his contribution had been futile.

When we ask someone to speak about their lived experiences, it's essential that we fully understand what we are asking of them, consider the aftermath and any effects on their welfare. Otherwise, we may be causing them harm, perhaps even exacerbating previous damage inflicted on them in healthcare settings.

I spoke to Eli Fitzgerald about this. As a young, neurodiverse, trans man living with HIV who works in the HIV sector, he is often asked to speak on panels about his lived experience. He told me that he has had some negative as well as positive experiences. One of the issues he highlighted was that 'people only hear what they want to hear'. He explained further that he was often asked to talk about his life experiences, but only within the limits of what was acceptable to them. He said, 'If they don't want to hear it, it doesn't matter if you shout.' He also described how being on a panel 'makes you feel like you are in a museum, like a talking statue. But this is my real life.'

Eli had some tips on how to improve the experience of patients who are asked to speak about their lived experiences. He advised acknowledging the power imbalances between the audience and the speaker and making efforts to ensure the speaker feels comfortable in the environment. He had experienced audiences who had made him feel that just because he had agreed to speak, they were entitled to ask him about any aspect of his life. Instead, he urged organisers to let speakers know that they could decline answering any questions they wanted, and to not feel guilty about it. Eli also talked about how the expectation from organisers is to always talk about trauma but being able to talk about joy makes the experience feel more balanced and less of a burden. He felt it was vital that speakers were not condescended to, and that medical jargon was avoided. Finally, he said that to get the best out of an invited patient speaker, he would recommend 'asking a question that matters' because then, 'you'll get an answer that matters'.

Valuing patient voice includes remuneration, which Eli also reiterated. Patients may be giving up other paid work to speak at an event, or they may not be able to work due to their illness, relying on sickness or disability benefits. It's therefore even more important that payment is offered from the start, as part of the invitation. This also means that the patient does not bear the burden and embarrassment of having to initiate the conversation. I have seen issues with unequitable remuneration on several occasions. A particularly memorable experience was being part of a paid advisory group focusing on improving care for women living with HIV. The group consisted of doctors, nurses, researchers, activists and women with HIV. It was fun to be part of, with everyone having the opportunity to offer their opinions and contribute. On the first day we made an agreement to share with each other how much we were being paid for the work. We quickly discovered that the women living with HIV were being offered considerably less than the clinicians and researchers. We felt this was unfair – after all, the group was convened to improve the lives of women living with HIV, so how could we tolerate those in the group having their lived experience valued less?

Together we asked the organisers to explain the disparity. They responded by saying they were compensating us for the wage that we would normally get in our day jobs – as medics and researchers, we would be earning more. While I understand the logic to this, I think it clearly demonstrates how patient voice and lived experience is not held to such a high regard as scientific expertise. The story has a happy ending – through collective bargaining, we ensured everyone in the group got paid the same as the medics. However, I suspect that such disparities are not rare.

Support may not just be monetary. In the podcast *Unlocking Us with Brené Brown* hosted by author Brené Brown, Tarana Burke, the founder of the MeToo movement, described how organisations asking survivors of sexual violence to speak about lived experiences could better support them.[8] She thought that this should go further than just payment; it should include pastoral support to deal with the trauma in their lives and to help them heal. We should consider this for patients too.

In the book *The Patient Revolution*, patient leader Ceinwen Giles summarises how requests for patients to speak are ill-considered, saying, 'I find there's a lot of take, take, take and not a lot of giving back.' She says that 'in healthcare, we have the idea that anyone can do it', asking, 'Why should I give up my time to come into some crappy building at 2 p.m. on a Wednesday where you get a bad cup of coffee?' She urges organisers to make the experience more pleasant with refreshments and acknowledgement of patients' time with gifts and other ways to thank them.[9]

Including patient voice and lived experience is essential in planning high-quality healthcare services and research, but we must make sure that when we ask patients to speak, we do not cause distress. This is not progress. In valuing the patient voice and truly listening, we must ethically consider the different ways in which we can support patients so their contribution is meaningful.

*

Hodan is a new consultant in respiratory medicine specialising in the treatment of asthma. She's really excited about stepping up into the role, having trained as a junior doctor for thirteen years, including completing a PhD. In her first week, Hodan meets the department's lead consultant to finalise her job plan, which will be a mix of clinics, ward rounds, on-call shifts and service development projects.

Towards the end of the meeting, her line manager mentions that the hospital management team have recently stated their intention to improve equality, diversity and inclusion (EDI) among the staff. As part of this they have convened a working group, who are in the process of writing a new policy and delivering teaching to staff. He suggests that Hodan should consider being a part of this group. It will be good experience for her and beneficial for their department to have her involved. EDI work wasn't something she had been significantly involved in before, but she is aware that new consultants are generally expected to say yes when asked to take on management work. So Hodan agrees, reasoning that it will be useful for her career development, but is apprehensive because her schedule is already packed. After the meeting she finds out that the other new consultant in the department, Nick, a white man, was not asked to contribute to the EDI group.

One year on, while preparing for her appraisal, Hodan reflects on how things have gone. She acknowledges the massive learning curve she's been through and is proud of what she's done, reinforced by the positive feedback from her colleagues. Hodan feels like a respected member of the department consultant team, which is incredibly satisfying. However, the EDI work has not been so fulfilling. She'd started with enthusiasm, having thought deeply about her own journey in the NHS, as a Muslim woman of Somali heritage, and the difficulties she had encountered along the way. She wanted to make sure others had it easier in the future. A large part of her role was to go out to different hospital departments and deliver training which focused on the importance of equality, diversity and inclusion for staff wellbeing, retention and ultimately patient care.

But more of these teaching experiences were negative rather than positive. Hodan had expected some resistance from audiences – talking about sexism, racism, ableism and other forms of oppression was always going to be uncomfortable, particularly for individuals confronting their biases for the first time. But what she hadn't expected was members of the audience directly challenging the evidence she was presenting, even though the statistics came from thorough research. She felt undermined and tired. The work was also time-intensive, leaving her unable to take on other work she was offered, such as being part of a medical advisory board for an asthma charity. She was gutted by this – it was something she was passionate about and would have been useful for her research and clinical career.

Additionally, many of the recommendations in the EDI strategy that Hodan and her colleagues had worked hard on had come back substantially watered down by senior hospital management. And at the launch, neither she nor her colleagues were asked to speak. Instead, it was the hospital senior managers who ended up getting the applause and attention for initiating the group, rather than those who did the work. Hodan was asked to be in the photo on the front cover of the policy, demonstrating the diversity of the EDI working group.

At Hodan's appraisal, her line manager was impressed with her achievements that year and encouraged her to apply to the local clinical excellence award scheme. This was for consultants who went above and beyond their job plan, for which they are awarded with a pay bonus. She was flattered by this, as she felt she had worked hard, so it was worth a try. But when she looked at the form, she realised that the EDI work did not fit any of the marking criteria so would not count in her favour. Ironically, if she'd had the time to take on the charity position, it would have.

Hodan felt frustrated that she had been asked to do the EDI role, feeling it was just because she was a Muslim woman of colour, not because she had expressed interest in the position before. Though she had given it her utmost attention and effort, it had been emotionally challenging and affected her self-confidence. Not only that, but it had also prevented her from working in other roles which she had more interest in; ones which would have been more beneficial for her career and could have led to a pay rise. And she was disappointed in the hospital leadership team, feeling that the EDI work they wanted was mere reputational management for the organisation, rather than resulting in any tangible actions to improve workplace conditions for minoritised staff. She resolved to say no to doing any further EDI work.

Hodan was doing 'diversity work'. Sara Ahmed says this can be work which is done to change an institution, or it can be work by those who do not 'quite inhabit the norms of an institution'. It is often people who are seen as 'the diversity' in institutions who are given the role of changing these norms, by becoming members of equality, diversity and inclusion groups. Ahmed goes on to say that 'embodying diversity can thus require additional work; the depletion of the energy of diversity workers is part of the embodied and institutional history of diversity'.[10] In other words, the burden of EDI work is often put on minoritised staff, as experienced by Hodan. Dr Uché Blackstock, a health equity expert, discusses this as well. Writing about why she left academic medicine, she said, 'I find it ironic that Black faculty members are unfairly tasked with the complex and overwhelming chore of remedying the structural outcomes of centuries of institutionalized racism that we did not create in the first place.'[11]

In the last few years, with increased focus on social inequality since the pandemic and the death of George Floyd, many organisations pledged to improve working conditions for minoritised staff. However, just three years on, commentators are critical of the efforts made so far. In an article for *Time*, journalist S. Mitra Kalita writes that, 'We're backsliding on this diversity thing' as many companies are having to lay off workers, the majority of whom are minoritised. She questions why this is and suggests it might be 'because the diversity efforts of the last three years have been largely cosmetic, performative, and perfunctory. We have barely begun to change the systems contributing to inequity.'[12] This shows some of what Hodan noticed – that hospital management wanted to be seen to be doing good EDI work, but when it came to actual change, they substantially weakened the recommendations.

Hodan's scenario shows how despite EDI work being essential for the healthcare workforce and patients, it is undervalued and uncompensated. These problems are preventable through proper investment to ensure staff are supported to do the work, crediting them for it, and making it part of the criteria for promotion. It's important that institutions like hospitals and universities consider the ethics of EDI work – as we've already seen there is a plethora of evidence to show that a more diverse and inclusive workforce leads to increased innovation, productivity and better outcomes for patients.

> 'Let me be devil's advocate.'
> 'I'm just asking a question.'
> 'I'm just offering an alternative explanation.'

These common statements often come up in Q&A discussions and teaching sessions. While they appear to be reasonable conversational norms, they are in fact a demand for more information from the speaker and indicate that perhaps an audience has not heard or fully considered the speaker's point of view or evidence. They are also examples of 'epistemic exploitation', a concept theorised by American philosopher Nora Berenstain in 2016.[13] She defines this as occurring when 'privileged persons compel marginalised persons to educate them about the nature of their oppression. It is marked by unrecognised, uncompensated, emotionally taxing, coerced epistemic labour.' This concept helps explain some of the difficulties that both Michael and Hodan encountered.

When Berenstain refers to 'epistemic labour', she is describing the work of producing and delivering knowledge. Examples of this include the talks I gave on racism and health, Hodan's EDI teaching and Michael's panel contribution. Berenstain writes about how this labour is often emotionally and cognitively demanding, but not acknowledged as work so it is often unsupported and unpaid.

Epistemic exploitation is widespread, but often under-recognised as it masquerades as a well-intentioned request to 'teach me about the nature of your oppression'. For example, a person of colour being asked by a white person to explain why an incident is racist. The white person asking this may be well-intentioned and want to understand racism better. However, this puts the burden of education on the person experiencing the racism, not the person privileged enough not to experience racism. The person of colour feels obliged to answer, to provide evidence of their experience. The white person asking the question is seen as being virtuous in wanting to know more. This happened to Hodan, who was asked to take on the EDI work in her department due to being a woman of colour – unlike her white male colleague, Nick, she was expected to do it and felt obliged to say yes. In this way, the work can sometimes feel coerced. Of course, this is not always the case – people from marginalised groups may want to educate others, but if so, they should be compensated for this.

Epistemic exploitation has several damaging effects. It results in unpaid labour and what Berenstain terms 'opportunity costs'. We can see this in Hodan's scenario where the work took a toll on her mentally and physically, and she did not receive credit for it. But it also meant that she missed out on opportunities to carry out the work she did want to do – volunteering for the asthma charity, which would be more useful for her long-term career and less emotionally taxing.

When she delivered the EDI awareness teaching to staff groups, Hodan was faced with challenges to the data she produced. Berenstain calls this 'default skepticism', where what the speaker says is dismissed by the more privileged audience, who question the veracity of the data ('how was this research carried out?') and may even question that the oppression has been demonstrated ('I don't think this shows that there is racism in the NHS'). Hodan felt undermined by the audiences in these sessions, which affected her self-confidence. Berenstain says such scepticism is another demand for more work – the audience is saying, 'I've asked you to educate me, but what you have said does not convince me. You need to tell me more, to convince me of your oppression.' This scepticism is also in its own way a privilege. If we don't experience a form of oppression, we can remain ignorant about it. For example, as an able-bodied person, I don't have to think about whether my workplace is accessible to colleagues.

Remaining wilfully ignorant about a matter allows people to

carry on profiting from unjust systems and to feel virtuous about it. In their book *How to Disagree,* philosophers Adam Ferner and Darren Chetty discuss how ignorance is not 'neutral – a void, where knowledge should be – it's an actively protected space'. They explain that the philosopher Plato described two forms of ignorance: single ignorance is 'a matter of knowing that you don't know something'; double ignorance 'involves not even being aware of what it is that you do not know'.[14] Often, double ignorance can be intentional, what is termed 'wilful ignorance'. This is where people can benefit by protecting themselves from uncomfortable truths. So, when an audience member intentionally pushes back at the evidence presented by an EDI speaker like Hodan, they are invested in maintaining their own wilful ignorance. Ferner and Chetty urge the reader to combat this. 'Rather than assuming we know all there is to know about a topic, it can be important to reflect on how knowledge and ignorance inform our deliberation. What is it that we are invested in not knowing? What might someone taking part in our conversation know that we don't?'

While epistemic exploitation was developed as a concept by Nora Berenstain, she acknowledges the work of the women of colour scholars before her who have described the phenomenon in different ways. For example, Toni Morrison, addressing Portland State University in 1975, said 'It's important, therefore, to know who the real enemy is, and to know the function, the very serious function of racism, which is distraction. It keeps you from doing your work. It keeps you explaining, over and over again, your reason for being.' She went on to say how this explaining is never enough: 'there will always be one more thing'.[15]

This well-known Morrison quote encapsulates how epistemic exploitation maintains structures of oppression by centring the needs and demands of privileged groups (here, white people), and exploiting the emotional and cognitive labour of members of marginalised groups (here, people of colour). These are also the people who benefit from the very systems of oppression (in this case, white supremacy) about which they demand to be educated.

One important feature of epistemic exploitation is how it allows the privileged to remain ignorant about oppression. Berenstain explains how marginalised people are often asked to produce resources such as books and talks to teach others on the nature of their oppression, but these are often dismissed and ignored by privileged people as not being genuine knowledge. This then allows them to say, 'If the resources aren't there, and you won't make them for me, then how can I be expected to learn?', providing an excuse to remain wilfully ignorant. This dismissal of the resources produced by marginalised groups is also a form of epistemic oppression – 'persistent epistemic exclusion that hinders one's contribution to knowledge production' theorised by philosopher Kristie Dotson, who we've encountered before.[16]

Injustice is furthered when we don't open our minds to new expert voices and consider arguments that are beyond and outside of our own. Listening, hearing and considering doesn't immediately mean agreeing: it's important we take our time to open ourselves up to knowledge we may not have previously heard before and give it time to sink in. Perhaps it might be enough to change your mind on a subject or open up a new avenue of interest, and there's real power in that.

When we ask people to speak on issues of equality, diversity and inclusion, what can we do to help make it less exploitative?

In the first instance, we must consider whether we need to put the burden of educating ourselves on others. Perhaps we can do our own research and reading? It is very likely that resources have been already created and are accessible. Berenstain discusses how people tend to hear and believe people who are like them, making the case for the more privileged groups to educate each other. For example, this could be white people teaching each other on racism. However, she warns that privileged people who do this teaching can develop an over-inflated sense of entitlement and arrogance that prevents them from continuing to listen to those who are marginalised. Instead, they believe *they* are the experts. Care must be taken to ensure they maintain their humility.

Secondly, we must acknowledge that we are asking people to do work and that this is often emotional and difficult. We must make sure people are credited appropriately, unlike Hodan and her colleagues who didn't get the recognition for their work on the EDI policy, the accolades going to the hospital management team. We should provide pastoral support such as opportunities to debrief if required. Just as when we ask patients to speak, this kind of work should be given parity with other kinds of work by remunerating people adequately.

Thirdly, we should consider our responsibilities when we are listening to someone speak. As we've seen in mine and Hodan's cases, audiences can be hostile to speakers. How can we avoid being confrontational? Ferner and Chetty advise that when we are in an audience ourselves, we should pause before we put up our hand to make a comment or ask a question and consider why. It may be for one of these reasons:

- Is it to fill a pregnant pause?
- Is it to hear the sound of our own voice?
- Do we believe we have a unique perspective on a particular issue?
- Is it more important for us to share our thoughts than to let someone else speak?[17]

This helps us to decide whether it is worthwhile still putting our hand up. They also advise a simple phrase that allows us to question the speaker in a way that is not confrontational. This is 'Can you tell me more?', which comes across as less judgemental and entitled than 'Why do you think this?' Session chairs should also consider that audiences may potentially be hostile to the speaker, and actively chair in a way that ensures that any attempts to silence or abuse the speaker are shut down quickly.

Finally, we must ensure that the emotional labour of diversity work results in concrete actions to make it worthwhile. It also avoids a more cosmetic approach which results in reputational management, rather than real institutional change.

Through my personal experience of doing diversity work, and through Michael's and Hodan's stories, I have shown that speaking up for the marginalised is difficult, emotional work and should be treated as such. By acknowledging this, we can listen in more ethical ways that make the speaker feel invigorated rather than drained. We also need to think about when we ourselves are asked to speak – can we do this in a more ethical manner?

*

When I've been asked to speak at an event or join a committee, it has usually felt like a compliment. It's nice to be asked and the experience is often positive. It's also a privilege to be asked, and as such, should be considered as one. When we say yes to such an offer, how can we ensure that we give the topic the attention that it deserves and speak in a more ethical way? In truth, this is something I never used to think about, instead feeling grateful for the opportunities coming my way. I have since learnt if I want to practice what I preach, then when I talk about equity, I must consider this issue.

Nowadays, I start by asking myself, 'Am I the right person to do this?' Just because I am a member of a marginalised group (women of colour), I think it's important to ask whether I am actually the right person to be contributing my knowledge in this forum. The politics of representation mean that to show diversity, institutions will ask for a representative from different minoritised groups to speak. But can we speak for everyone in our group? The answer is of course not, and nor should we. I cannot speak for every upper caste Hindu, middle-class woman brought up in Essex of Indian heritage, let alone every woman of colour. Diversity also means a diversity of opinions and so people in marginalised groups will have very different opinions about the nature of their oppression and what to do about it. The philosopher Linda M. Alcoff urges that we should aim for 'the practice of speaking with and to rather than speaking for others' as this will reduce the possibilities of misrepresentation and increasing our own 'authority and privilege'.[18]

Just because I am a member of a minoritised group doesn't mean I will experience a particular oppression. For example, I may be asked to join a working group focusing on how to reduce so-called honour-based abuse, because I am a British Asian woman. Yes, I may understand some Asian cultures better than the white people in the group, but I cannot speak for a British Asian woman who has been directly affected by so-called honour-based abuse. I therefore need to think about my own limitations when agreeing to speak or be part of a committee. I also need to recognise that other people may put a heavy weight on what I say, just because I am British Asian. They may credit me with a credibility excess, believing I know more than I actually do. This means it's even more important that I think about what I am saying and whether I am the right person to take such an opportunity.

The American philosopher Olúfẹ́mi O. Táíwò has written about this issue in his 2022 book, *Elite Capture*.[19] He talks about how if you're present where these conversations are happening, then you hold privilege, which he terms 'in the room privilege'. We need to think about who's not in the room, and how we can strive to bring them into conversations – these truly are the unheard voices that we need to hear. He discusses the current shift to 'centre the most marginalised' or 'listen to the most affected', a form of what he calls 'deference politics'. This is sometimes called 'passing the mic' – giving the people most affected by the oppression the chance to speak. This sounds like a good thing to do, but Táíwò points out the problems with it, writing that 'Instead, "centering the most marginalized" in my experience has usually meant handing conversational authority and attentional goods to whoever is already in the room and appears to fit a social category associated with some form of oppression – regardless of what they have or have not actually experienced, or what they do or do not actually know about the matter at hand.'

Táíwò uses the example of Black people in the US in academic spaces being asked to talk about increased rates of incarceration for Black people. He says that although the Black person in the academic space may be better placed to speak on this than the white people there, they remain privileged as they are already in the room. He emphasises that this type of deference politics is often well-intentioned. However, he explains that 'the facts that explain who ends up in what room shape our world much more powerfully than the squabbles for comparative prestige between people who have already made it inside.' The facts that need changing are the societal processes that cause these inequities. He goes on to say: 'The fact that incarcerated people cannot participate in academic discussions about freedom is intimately related to the fact that they are physically locked in cages.' So, when we are asked to speak as a member of a minoritised group, it's important that we know our limitations. We can also encourage the organisers to invite other people from our group, so we are not tokens and that there is a diversity of thought.

I also ask myself, 'Am I appropriately crediting the people that I have gained my knowledge from?' We all get ideas from other people, and we build on these to create our own insights and knowledge. This is an important part of advancing knowledge. However, people from marginalised groups may be more likely to be asked to share their knowledge and may feel they are expected to. Dr Autumn Asher BlackDeer, a decolonial scholar-activist from the Southern Cheyenne Nation in North America tweeted about this. 'Imagine if we charged for every time someone wanted to "pick our brain" (aka provide free emotional labor and reassure them as their friendly local marginalized pal that they're surely not racist/homophobic/ableist/etc). Like we could all retire tomorrow.'[20] This tweet highlights the invisible work that is often unacknowledged and not credited. This has happened to me on several occasions, where I have seen people's published work or talks building on ideas of mine, but not referencing me. This may not sound important, but citations are an important measure of academic success. Scholars are scored on it and it is used as criteria to show how much impact your research and thinking has, something that affects promotion and pay.

Ethical citational practice also includes thinking about *who* you are citing. Sara Ahmed has written about this extensively. She gives an example of how when she was asked to contribute to a sociology course, she found the core reading was written by men. When she highlighted this, she says, 'The course convener implied that that was simply a reflection of the history of the discipline. Well: this is a very selective history! The reproduction of a discipline can be the reproduction of these techniques of selection, ways of making certain bodies and thematics core to the discipline, and others not even part.'[21] Ahmed advises that we can and should try and cite people whose voices are less heard, or who may have been overlooked. African American scholar Audre Lorde wrote about this too: 'And where the words of women are crying to be heard, we must each of us recognize our responsibility to seek those words out, to read them and share them and examine them in their pertinence to our lives.'[22] Ethical citational practice can be used when we speak and when we write, so we acknowledge the work of others which has guided our own, and do our best to amplify marginalised scholars. For me, this is important, and something I've tried to demonstrate in this book, though I am aware there is always room for improvement. I know my voice is one among many who have explored and brought forward knowledge on these subjects, and while I believe I'm bringing new ideas to this conversation, I know I've been inspired by so many others.

When I am asked to speak or be part of a committee, I consider my obligations to myself, an important form of self-care that I recommend to everyone and something that can be applied to almost anything. I ask myself:

- Do I have time to do this?
- Do I have the energy and emotional reserve?
- What will I need to give up in order to do this?
- What will I receive in compensation? (This just may be the feeling of having contributed to something worthwhile, but this is an active choice on my part; I do not feel coerced or exploited. I am aware that being able to work for free is a privilege that many don't have.)

Since my revelation about the emotional and unacknowledged labour I had been carrying out during the first years of the COVID-19 pandemic, I'm also now much better at saying no than I used to be. This has been beneficial for my mental and physical health. It has also given me the opportunity to recommend and support other people to do the work, those who may want a step-up, career wise. It means I can try and lift up others, a form of practising what I preach when it comes to equity work.

*

Audre Lorde's quote, 'Caring for myself is not self-indulgence, it is self-preservation, and that is an act of political warfare'[23] is widely used to emphasise the importance of self-care. While often understood to be about looking after ourselves as individuals, it can also mean self-care in communities. As a global community of people striving to improve healthcare, we as patients, healthcare workers and researchers should concentrate on looking after each other when it comes to listening and speaking up. It's only by doing this that we will hear what needs to be said, however uncomfortable this may be.

Summary: How we can listen more ethically as a community

- When we ask people (including patients) to speak about their lived experiences:
  - Acknowledge power imbalances and strive to ensure the speaker feels comfortable and supported.
  - Avoid asking the speaker to just talk about trauma. If they do, ensure there is pastoral support available at the time and afterwards.
  - Recognise this is epistemic work, of equal value to other expertise, and remunerate adequately and equitably.
  - Make the experience more pleasant – refreshments and environment can all help with this.
  - Instigate change and involve them in this process.

- When we ask people to do equality, diversity and inclusion work:
  - Ensure this is properly resourced and prioritised in the institution.
  - Recognise this is epistemic work and remunerate appropriately.
  - Make sure the work leads to transformational change, not just reputational management.
  - Listen to them with an open mind and understand that if you feel uncomfortable by what they say, this is normal. This work is meant to challenge us, so we can feel galvanised to challenge injustice. If you want to question the speaker, consider asking 'Can you tell me more?', which comes across as non-confrontational.
  - Don't always expect the person in the team with lived experience of marginalisation to do EDI work.
  - Challenge your own blind spots and think about what knowledge you are invested in not knowing.

- ○ Take on responsibility for educating yourself – find out what learning resources are already available and use them.

- When we are asked to speak:
  - ○ Ask yourself if you are the right person to speak at this moment.
  - ○ Ensure you are not a token – could the organisers invite other speakers to provide not only diversity of identity, but diversity of thought?
  - ○ Consider the politics of citation – are you crediting everyone whose work you are using or building on, and are you drawing on the work of a large range of people?
  - ○ What are your obligations to yourself if you accept the opportunity – do you have the time and energy to do this? What will you get for doing this work, and what are you giving up?

Conclusion

Are We Ready to Listen?

When I was younger, I lost my voice.

I was a cheeky child, often told off by my parents for being naughty, and I had a talent for annoying my older sister. But my school reports told a different story. Every year my teachers complained that I was 'too shy and needed to speak up more'. Why this marked difference between the 'school me' and the 'home me'? It wasn't the schoolwork that was putting me off – I got good marks. At some point I learnt to keep quiet, work hard and not stand out.

I wonder if this silencing of my voice coincided with the loss of my mother tongue, Marathi. When we moved from India to England, I was only two years old and couldn't speak English. My parents, like many other migrant parents at the time, were keen for us to fit in. We mainly spoke English at home. We'd go back to Mumbai for long summer holidays every year, where I'd spend hours playing with my cousins, running up and down the stairs of the six-storey building my extended family lived in, and playing cricket in the car park. On returning to school, my headteacher would tell my parents that I had come back with an Indian accent and encourage me to lose it. When my headteacher pointed this out, I suddenly became aware of how I spoke. I started to be more careful with what I said and how I said it. I was scared of getting things wrong and stopped putting my hand up in class. I had been effectively quietened. I adapted by being shy at school and made up for this by being loud at home. Now, while I can understand Marathi to a child's level, I can no longer speak it. As an adult this feels like a significant loss.

I didn't just lose my first language, I lost relationships. While my relatives could all speak English to varying degrees, it was harder to speak with my grandparents as they got older. We'd communicate with hugs and kisses and when they'd speak Marathi to me, I replied in English. I became apprehensive at even attempting Marathi, nervous of being laughed at and ashamed of this fear. This lack of confidence in languages remains with me now. It also made me feel less like I belonged – I couldn't see a future where living and working in Mumbai was a possibility.

Another headteacher helped me find my voice. I went to a selective girl's school where we were taught to believe we could do anything we wanted to, if we worked hard enough. My headteacher embodied this: for us she was a vision of female success – young, fiercely intelligent and glamorous. To ensure she knew the names of all the pupils in the school, she taught year 7 pupils 'Oral English'. These were sessions to help us gain confidence in public speaking. Looking back, this was well thought out – she knew that as women we would have to make an extra effort to be heard and wanted us to be prepared for it. I can remember she once divided us into small groups where we took it in turns to facilitate the group in carrying out a task. When it was my turn, she hovered nearby and afterwards told me that I was a 'natural-born leader'. I couldn't believe it! No one had ever recognised that in me before. It instilled in me a little seed of confidence – the hope that one day I would feel less scared to make my presence known.

It hasn't been a straightforward journey. There've been times in my life when I wish I'd spoken up more as a patient and as a doctor. I've been a very junior doctor on chronically understaffed and possibly unsafe rotas; I've been bullied by senior colleagues and struggled to stick up for myself. Each time this happened, it ate away at my self-confidence and I felt demoralised. But the times I have felt more able to speak up have been when advocating for others. I'm proud to say that over the years through my work with minoritised colleagues and patients, and my own experiences as a patient, I have found my voice again. I'm empowered to use it to challenge injustices in healthcare. I want to encourage others to speak up for themselves and this book is part of that. As I've shown, silencing is depressingly common in all aspects of medicine, but I believe that by supporting those who are unheard, we will create a healthcare system that is safer and more equitable for everyone.

I've used my own and others' experiences of being a patient to demonstrate how, when patients are repeatedly not listened to, dismissed, or disbelieved, this leads to silencing. I have shown how epistemic injustice is more likely to happen to people who have long had their social identity negatively stereotyped, including women, people of colour, LGBTQ+ people, the very old and the very young, disabled people, the working classes and people from religious minorities. This can have a damaging impact on their health including delayed diagnosis or misdiagnosis, inappropriate treatment and even death. I've held a mirror up to myself and my profession to understand why doctors find it hard to listen to patients. Not only are healthcare systems not designed to encourage or incentivise listening, but medical education teaches doctors to doubt patients and imbues them with a sense of hubris – this is a wall to better understanding. From our time as students, we are taught to keep a distance from patients, to listen selectively and with a degree of scepticism. This outlook is even ingrained in the language of medicine and contributes to power imbalances in the doctor–patient relationship. I've also found that this issue strikes deep into the heart of our profession, making us question our role as doctors. Are we fixers, or healers? How do we balance the need to have boundaries with being open to hearing everything patients tell us? The answers to these questions are hard to pin down, but I think by understanding the value of listening and providing opportunities for debrief and supervision, we become better doctors. Creating boundaries is a hard task, one that comes with practice and thought, but I hope I've given some insight into how it is possible. There is greatness that comes with real human connection, and its value needs to be reinforced in healthcare.

It's true that patients are adversely affected both directly and in-directly when doctors don't listen to each other. Minoritised doctors often advocate for minoritised patients and the health conditions that affect them, and when these doctors are not listened to or are made to feel like they don't belong, it creates a culture of exclusion. When doctors aren't representing people of all backgrounds or they are only considering health issues that impact the Western world, then we are not a truly equal and equitable healthcare system. Marginalised voices, and the conditions they speak of, are important and we need marginalised researchers to be taken seriously and considered credible knowledge producers. If we don't do this, I have shown how it can lead to gaps in our collective medical know-ledge. This has happened historically on a global scale because of the enduring impact of colonialism, and the power hierarchies it enforced have led to the silencing of researchers and communities in the Global South.

For the last three decades, the dominant paradigm for medicine has been evidence-based. While there is no doubt that it has made clinical practice safer and more efficient, it has privileged certain types of medical evidence over others. Though the promotion of scientific objectivity helped cement medicine as a profession, it has led to the systematic downgrading of patient voice, particularly in health conditions for which there are fewer signs and tests. It has meant these conditions have been deprioritised for research and health policy, marginalising those suffering from them. This has resulted in care being lacking in our healthcare services. This systematic denial of the human, the subjective and the pastoral, has led to patients working collectively to be heard. Patients shouldn't have to fight for attention, and while there will always be a need for prioritisation in the medical world, there also needs to be an openness to diversify the conditions receiving focus. There are patients who are underserved, and their lives should hold value no matter how complex or unclear their conditions may be, and no matter what background they come from.

We need to be gentle with each other when we do take the time to speak up, and be mindful when we listen. It is about giving value to the perspectives of those who often aren't compensated, and being self-aware when we don't need to be the loudest voice in the room. Ethical listening creates greater justice in all areas of work and life, but in the space of health it is even more pressing to get it right. Patients come to us vulnerable, scared and hopeful and seek our advice on conditions that are intimate, distressing and incredibly urgent for them, so giving them our full attention should be the standard. Such a standard has slipped, and this is what I've been addressing. I've suggested solutions – pragmatic and clear ways to improve listening, including empowering patients to be better prepared to speak up for themselves. I give this with the caveat that the onus of change should not be on them, but on healthcare systems – however, while they are imperfect, developing health literacy can help. I've given my advice on individual and systematic ways in which bias and discrimination can be addressed in patient care and in the workforce, and I've given my prescription for recognising the value of listening as being therapeutic in itself. We can provide healthcare that is more holistic, and doing so can be beneficial for us as doctors. Undoubtedly, doctors will need support with this, and introducing supervision and mentoring and reducing the conditions for burnout may help. In time, I would hope that the silencing, which has created that active and reinforced void which should never have become a medical practice, is filled with human connection.

To make this change requires an intentional shift in power, from the medical establishment to patients; from the marginalised to the privileged. This means some people will need to give up their power and persuading them of this will not be easy. The philosopher Kate Manne writes in her book *Down Girl: The Logic of Misogyny* how privilege is often 'well-defended and difficult to challenge', as people who hold it are often unwilling to let it go. This is made more difficult as the privilege is often invisible to the people who hold it. She warns that 'dismantling them may feel not only like a comedown, but also an injustice, to the privileged. They will tend to feel flattened, rather than merely levelled, in the process.'[1]

An example of this was in December 2022, when an NHS trust advertised for a Director of Lived Experience. The salary of £110,000–£115,000 a year was commensurate with other executive-level posts. The role included responsibility for amplifying the voice of service users at all levels of the organisation and promoting co-production projects (which involved patients and the public in their design). It stated that the aim of the post was to facilitate cultural change to ensure best practice around shared decision-making with patients. Despite many supporters from the medical profession, it did have its detractors on social media. It was criticised for being too 'gold standard' – if there wasn't enough funding for basics like sufficient staff and beds, then how could so much money be spent on this? There has also been a backlash against equality, diversity and inclusion (EDI) work in the NHS, with some newspapers commenting that it was too expensive. Inflammatory headlines like 'NHS spends more than £8.2m on "woke warriors" in diversity jobs' were printed.[2] This despite EDI roles only accounting for 0.03 per cent of NHS jobs. My response to such criticism is that listening to patients and improving EDI at every level is fundamental. If we can get healthcare right for the most marginalised in society, everyone will benefit. We need to incorporate these values into the core of everything we do, and right from the start of training.

At the time of writing, there has been a high-profile case of a neonatal nurse accused of murdering babies under her care at an NHS trust in England. More facts about the case are emerging, but it's apparent that several of her colleagues, including consultants, had repeatedly raised their suspicions about her to hospital management, but had been dismissed. This has prompted a widespread conversation about how there is a culture in the NHS of reputational management above patient safety. There are many instances of frontline staff who have reported their concerns and been ignored, or even suppressed. Alison Leary, a professor of healthcare and workforce modelling, has written about the lack of a robust safety infrastructure in health organisations and the emphasis on individuals to speak up. Instead, she says, 'When workers are listened to and constructive dissent is encouraged and normalised, along with the reporting of incidents, there is little need for whistle-blowing. A workforce that must resort to whistle-blowing is a symptom of poor safety culture.'[3] This reiterates the point that we cannot rely on people being brave and speaking up, we must learn to listen better and make it safe for people to voice their concerns.

Governments are responsible for providing the resources and infrastructure to ensure healthcare services meet demand and are safe. It's essential that they listen to healthcare staff and patients, but this doesn't seem to be the case in England where the NHS is in a perpetual state of crisis.[4] Waiting lists for elective care have risen and patient satisfaction is low. The workforce is demonstrating its unhappiness with several professional groups holding strikes to protest pay and work conditions. These strikes are unprecedented and reflect the fear that reduced recruitment and retention of staff will leave the NHS even more under-resourced than it is now. A General Medical Council Workforce survey in 2022 found that doctors reported increasing workloads, bullying and discrimination, sick leave due to stress and burnout. This was impacting patient care.[5] Figures comparing overall spend on healthcare between countries shows that the UK is below average in Europe for funding, numbers of beds and doctors per person. If the government genuinely wants an NHS that is safe and sustainable then it is going to need to listen to its stakeholders and commit to more investment.

Health is much more than just healthcare. Government policies can have a huge impact on the wider determinants of health. Since the global financial crash in 2007–8, policies of austerity have halted and even reversed progress in health outcomes. In 2020, 'Health Equity in England: The Marmot Review 10 Years On' was published, which found that progress in health outcomes had halted and even reversed in some regions.[6] Specifically, it reported that a greater number of people spend more of their lives in poor health, improvements to life expectancy have stalled and even declined for the poorest women, and there is worsening inequality by region. This includes the health gap growing between deprived areas in the north and prosperous areas in the south-east of England. The review concluded that this was a result of austerity policies, which had, among other impacts, increased child poverty, homelessness and food insecurity. Research shows that there is a direct link between poverty and health and this starts from an early age – adverse experiences in childhood affect people's health as adults. At a minimum, governments need to listen to groups campaigning against child poverty and to implement policies that lift more families above the breadline. In my daily work, I am lucky to be able to refer patients who are struggling to charities like Positive East, the Terrence Higgins Trust and The Food Chain[7-9] who help with accessing food, emergency funds, housing and benefits. The need for these has increased in recent years and I fervently hope for a time where I have fewer patients who require these services.

Governments also decide on laws which can affect the human rights and consequently the health of the most marginalised. For example, the increasingly hostile environment for immigrants deters people from accessing healthcare. This means they don't attend services until they are gravely ill. I've seen this happen first hand with patients who have literally collapsed into the emergency department, so unwell they have required intensive care for weeks. Apart from the moral implications of anti-immigrant policies, keeping people away from healthcare services is a false economy. Treating conditions early on or even preventing them is much more cost-effective.[10] People who are healthy are able to work, which means they can be productive members of society. Laws around the world criminalising LGBTQ+ people are similarly damaging to health. They are more likely to acquire HIV, because they cannot access sexual health education or prevention tools.[11] Although we do not yet know the full impact of the reversal of Roe vs Wade in the United States, we can predict that ending the constitutional right to abortion will mean that desperate women will again have to seek the services of unsafe, backstreet providers.[12] Increasing conflict and the effects of climate change are having a huge impact on people's health and governments have a key part to play with these.

Doctors need to make changes, but governments must also recognise the significant role they have in keeping their population healthy. To do this, they must listen to us all. I'm optimistic that change is coming and, in some cases, has even started. There are many inspiring individuals, groups and movements that are doing work to rehumanise healthcare. I've written about some of them in this book and there are many more. I think it's important to look at change and progress to sustain our motivation for making the world better, so I want to leave you with some examples.

Martha's Rule

In Chapter 1, I wrote about Martha Mills, who heartbreakingly died at the age of just thirteen with sepsis following an injury to her pancreas from a bicycle accident. Despite her parents raising concerns several times about sepsis, they were ignored by the medical team. The coroner reviewing her case stated that Martha was likely to have survived if she had been moved to intensive care earlier. Since her death, her parents Merope Mills and Paul Laity have successfully campaigned for Martha's Rule, which will include giving patients and their loved ones a right to a second senior medical opinion.[13] The government in England have said that they are committed to implementing the scheme and I believe this will be a big step towards putting some of the power back in patients' hands.

Advances in the treatment of sickle cell disease

As we've seen, sickle cell disease is the most common genetic condition around the world, but it has been neglected with regards to patient care and treatment. Encouragingly, progress is happening, and a gene therapy called Casgevy has been licensed. It works by using a gene-editing technique called CRISPR (genetic scissors) to edit the gene that causes sickle cell disease. This would allow the body to produce normal haemoglobin and has the potential to cure people and prevent much suffering.[14] However, its current cost is more than $2 million per treatment, which will limit its usefulness for now.

Awareness of perimenopause

Perimenopause is the stage before menopause, when periods stop. It can last several years as the ovaries gradually stop working. While this is a normal process associated with ageing, for some women it can come with debilitating symptoms such as hot flushes, tiredness, vaginal dryness, anxiety and insomnia. This has been under-recognised in the past by doctors, and women have often had their symptoms dismissed or attributed to other causes. In the last few years there has been a huge push to raise awareness of this so that women can access support to lessen their symptoms.[15] Encouragingly this has come from all sides – women experiencing symptoms, celebrity endorsers and concerned doctors and researchers. It is a great example of collaborative work to deliver real change.

Better access to new drugs for tuberculosis

Bedaquiline is a new drug to treat multidrug-resistant tuberculosis, an increasingly common condition around the world, affecting marginalised populations. However, due to its price it has been out of reach for many people who have needed it. Thanks to patient activism, an agreement with the pharmaceutical company Johnson & Johnson, who produce the drug, has been made, halving its price from $289 to $130 for a six-month course. It has been estimated that this will allow 51,000 more people to be treated.[16]

Health justice

Health justice, as described by the organisation Healing Justice Ldn, is an inspiring movement 'that seeks to name and disrupt the conditions that produce mass ill health and suffering'.[17] It looks at health at a broader level, rather than just the concern of individuals who need to be treated in a healthcare service. Healthcare is seen as something that 'should be proactively embedded on a structural and community level'.[18] This includes addressing the social and political determinants of health such as poverty, conflict and climate change. This makes a lot of sense to me – if we can prevent people from getting unwell in the first place, this would have a bigger impact than any advances in healthcare or treatment.

Deep medicine

This recognises that humans are part of an ecosystem, and as such our destinies are combined with that of the earth. By listening to the needs of our planet, such as addressing climate change, we can all be healthier. In *Inflamed: Deep Medicine and the Anatomy of Injustice*, Raj Patel and Rupa Marya explain this further, writing how humans have evolved alongside animals, plants and other organisms in the world. They say, 'the study of ecology is becoming indispensable to the study of medicine because humans are not just a single animal, but a multitude, an ecology of beings living on us, in us, and around us.'[19] Deep medicine is not just a theory, it is being put into practice, albeit with different names. In Scotland, for example, it is called 'realistic medicine'. Scotland's chief medical officer, Sir Gregor Smith, has published his intent to move away from an industrialised, transactional model of medicine to one that is person-focused. Its core elements are being human; value-based health and care; turning the tide on health inequalities; and climate and health. Smith says that the emphasis should shift from 'what often feels like industrial care performed by transactional technicians' to delivering 'the careful and kind care that will create the fairer, more sustainable system that we all wish to see'.[20] I find this incredibly heartening. I would like to work in such a system and as I get older, I would like to be cared for in such a system.

These stories are intended to give you hope, and for me, they demonstrate what happens when we listen and connect.

Though positive change is happening and maintaining a hopeful outlook is important, we also need to stay grounded in reality, and the reality is that people have gone unheard in medicine for a very long time. We are a long way from health justice. Significant change is needed and this needs to come from everyone – this includes patients, healthcare staff, researchers, funders, policymakers, politicians and the general public. This book is one step in the journey and I hope that I have inspired you to be part of this change, to challenge injustice, even if it is in a small way. I may have encouraged you to speak up for those who are marginalised, or to speak up for yourself. My main aim is that you feel better able to listen – to think about whose voices have been silenced and consider who isn't 'in the room'. How can you support their voices to be heard? This could range from accompanying a friend to their doctor's appointment to provide moral support, to passing an opportunity onto someone else so they have a turn to speak, to voting in the interests of the most marginalised. If you are a healthcare professional, how can you incorporate better listening into your practice on a daily basis? If you work in policy or research, how can you work with communities to make sure their views are heard?

Paul Farmer, co-founder of the global health organisation Partners in Health, said 'If access to health care is considered a human right, who is considered human enough to have that right?'[21] By working together to ensure those who are silenced get heard, we can have a healthcare system that treats everyone with dignity.

Are you ready to listen?

Bibliography and Endnotes

Introduction

1. Williams S. 'How Serena Williams Saved Her Own Life'. *Elle* magazine, 5 April 2022. https://www.elle.com/life-love/a39586444/how-serena-williams-saved-her-own-life/ [accessed 15 February 2024].

2. Ockenden D. 'The Ockenden Report'. Department of Health and Social Care independent maternity review. gov.uk. 30 March 2022. https://www.gov.uk/government/publications/final-report-of-the-ockenden-review/ockenden-review-summary-of-findings-conclusions-and-essential-actions [accessed 15 February 2024].

3. MBRRACE-UK. 'Saving Lives, Improving Mothers' Care'. 2021. https://www.npeu.ox.ac.uk/assets/downloads/mbrrace-uk/reports/maternal-report-2021/MBRRACE-UK_Maternal_Report_2021_-_Lay_Summary_v10.pdf [accessed 15 February 2024].

4. Birthrights UK. 'Systemic racism, not broken bodies'. 2022. https://www.birthrights.org.uk/campaigns-research/racial-injustice/ [accessed 15 February 2024].

5. Centers for Disease Control and Prevention. 'Maternal mortality rates in the United States'. 2020. https://www.cdc.gov/nchs/data/hestat/maternal-mortality/2020/maternal-mortality-rates-2020.htm [accessed 15 February 2024].

6. Leal M.D.C. *et al*. 'The color of pain: racial iniquities in prenatal care and childbirth in Brazil'. *Cad Saude Publica*, 24 July 2017;33Suppl 1(Suppl 1):e00078816. Portuguese, English. doi: 10.1590/0102-311X00078816. PMID: 28746555.

7. Draper E.S. *et al*. on behalf of the MBRRACE-UK Collaboration. 'Perinatal Mortality Surveillance, UK Perinatal Deaths for Births from January to December 2021: State of the Nation Report'. Leicester: The Infant Mortality and Morbidity Studies, Department of Population Health Sciences, University of Leicester, 2023.

8. The Sands Listening Project. 'Learning from the experiences of Black and Asian bereaved parents'. Sands. https://www.sands.org.uk/get-involved/get-involved-research/sands-listening-project-learning-experiences-black-and-asian [accessed 15 February 2024].

9. Meghani S.H., Byun E., Gallagher R.M. 'Time to take stock: a meta-analysis and systematic review of analgesic treatment disparities for pain in the United States'. *Pain Med*, 2012;13(2):150-174. doi:10.1111/j.1526-4637.2011.01310.

10. Hoffman K.M., Trawalter S., Axt J.R., Oliver M.N. 'Racial bias in pain assessment and treatment recommendations, and false beliefs about biological differences between blacks and whites'. *Proc Natl Acad Sci USA*, 2016;113(16):4296–4301. doi:10.1073/pnas.1516047113.

11. Hoffmann D.E. and Tarzian A.J. 'The Girl Who Cried Pain: A Bias Against Women in the Treatment of Pain'. 2001. Available at SSRN: https://ssrn.com/abstract=383803 or http://dx.doi.org/10.2139/ssrn.383803.

12. Chen E.H., Shofer F.S., Dean A.J. *et al.* 'Gender disparity in analgesic treatment of emergency department patients with acute abdominal pain'. *Acad Emerg Med*, 2008;15(5):414-418. doi:10.1111/j.1553-2712.2008.00100.x.

13. Harvard Health Blog. 'Women and pain: Disparities in experience and treatment'. Harvard Health Publishing, 9 October 2017. https://www.health.harvard.edu/blog/women-and-pain-disparities-in-experience-and-treatment-2017100912562 [accessed 15 February 2024].

14. Williams S. (n 1).

15. Roy A. Sydney Peace Prize Lecture: 'Peace & The New Corporate Liberation Theology'. Sydney Peace Foundation, 3 November 2004. https://sydneypeacefoundation.org.au/peace-prize-recipients/2004-arundhati-roy/ [accessed 15 February 2024].

16. Arcaya M.C., Arcaya A.L., Subramanian S.V. 'Inequalities in health: definitions, concepts, and theories'. *Glob Health Action*, 2015;8:27106. 24 June 2015. doi:10.3402/gha.v8.27106.

17. Watt L. 'Gonorrhoea in Manchester. Incidence of Repeated Infections'. *Brit J Vener Dis*, 1958. 34, 9 PMID: 13570629.

18. UK Health Security Agency. 'Sexually transmitted infections and screening for chlamydia in England: 2022 report'. gov.uk, 2023. https://www.gov.uk/government/statistics/sexually-transmitted-infections-stis-annual-data-tables/sexually-transmitted-infections-and-screening-for-chlamydia-in-england-2022-report [accessed 10 April 2024].

19. Dhairyawan R., Okhai H., Hill T., Sabin C.A. UK Collaborative HIV Cohort (UK CHIC) study. 'Differences in HIV clinical outcomes amongst heterosexuals in the United Kingdom by ethnicity'. *AIDS*, 2021;35(11):1813–1821. doi:10.1097/QAD.0000000000002942.

20. All Party Parliamentary Group on HIV and AIDS. '"Nothing about us without us": Addressing the needs of Black, Asian and Minority Ethnic communities in relation to HIV in the UK'. 14 April 2022. https://www.appghivaids.org.uk/news [accessed 15 February 2024].

21. Marmot M., Allen J., Boyce T. *et al.* 'Health Equity in England: The Marmot Review 10 Years On'. London: Institute of Health Equity, 2010.

22. Wade C., Malhotra A.M., McGuire P., Vincent C., Fowler A. 'Action on patient safety can reduce health inequalities'. *BMJ*, 2022; 376:e067090. doi:10.1136/bmj-2021-067090.

23. Bachmann C. and Gooch B. 'LGBT Health in Britain'. Stonewall, November 2018. https://www.stonewall.org.uk/lgbt-britain-health [accessed 15 February 2024].

24. Saunders C.L., Berner A., Lund J., Mason A.M., Oakes-Monger T., Roberts M., Smith J., Duschinsky R. 'Demographic characteristics, long-term health conditions and healthcare experiences of 6333 trans and non-binary adults in England: nationally representative evidence from the 2021 GP Patient Survey'. *BMJ Open*, 2 February 2023; 13(2):e068099. doi: 10.1136/bmjopen-2022-068099. PMID: 36731935; PMCID: PMC9895920.

25. Chang E.S., Kannoth S., Levy S., Wang S.Y., Lee J.E., Levy B.R. 'Global reach of ageism on older persons' health: A systematic review'. *PLoS One*, 15 January 2020; 15(1):e0220857. doi: 10.1371/journal.pone.0220857. PMID: 31940338; PMCID: PMC6961830.

26. NHS Race and Health Observatory. 'We Deserve Better: Ethnic minorities with a learning difficulty and access to healthcare'. July 2023. https://www.nhsrho.org/research/review-into-factors-that-contribute-towards-inequalities-in-health-outcomes-faced-by-those-with-a-learning-disability-from-a-minority-ethnic-community/ [accessed 15 February 2024].

27. Kapadia D., Zhang J., Salway S. *et al.* 'Ethnic inequalities in healthcare: a rapid evidence review'. NHS Race and Health Observatory, June 2021. https://www.nhsrho.org/research/ethnic-inequalities-in-healthcare-a-rapid-evidence-review-2/ [accessed 15 February 2024].

28. Allington D., McAndrew S., Duffy B. *et al.* 'Trust and experiences of National Health Service healthcare do not fully explain demographic disparities in coronavirus vaccination uptake in the UK: a cross-sectional study'. *BMJ Open*, 2022;12:e053827. doi: 10.1136/bmjopen-2021-053827.

29. Luther King Jr. M. Presentation at the Second National Convention of the Medical Committee for Human Rights, Chicago, 25 March 1966.

30. Fricker M. *Epistemic Injustice: Power and the Ethics of Knowing*. Oxford: Oxford University Press, 2007.

1: Dismissed

1. Telfer C. 'We need less "sickle cell warriors" and more allies'. Wellcome Collection, 17 April 2023. https://wellcomecollection.org/articles/ZCo8WBQ AANdrVsZu [accessed 15 February 2024].

2. APPG on Sickle Cell and Thalassaemia and the Sickle Cell Society. The Sickle Cell Society, November 2021. https://www.sicklecellsociety.org/wp-content/uploads/2021/11/No-Ones-Listening-Final.pdf [accessed 15 February 2024].

3. Ormiston S. 'Sickle cell sufferer, 46, left screaming in agony died after hospital neglect'. MyLondon, 1 October 2021. https://www.mylondon.news/news/sickle-cell-sufferer-singer-songwriter-21730986 [accessed 15 February 2024].

4. 'Mother launches legal investigation into son's sickle cell death at Northwick Park Hospital'. Leigh Day, 22 December 2021. https://www.leighday.co.uk/news/news/2021-news/mother-launches-legal-investigation-into-son-s-sickle-cell-death-at-northwick-park-hospital/ [accessed 15 February 2024].

5. 'Inquest finds failure to appreciate sickle cell crisis symptoms in the death of 21-year-old Evan Nathan Smith'. Leigh Day, 6 April 2021. https://www.leigh-day.co.uk/latest-updates/news/2021-news/inquest-finds-failure-to-appreciate-sickle-cell-crisis-symptoms-in-the-death-of-21-year-old-evan-nathan-smith/ [accessed 15 February 2024].

6. Mathers M. 'Death of sickle cell patient who rang 999 from hospital bed could have been prevented, coroner says'. *The Independent*, 8 April 2021. https://www.independent.co.uk/news/uk/home-news/evan-nathan-smith-death-sickle-cell-b1827443.html [accessed 11 April 2024].

7. APPG on Sickle Cell. (n 2).

8. Ibid.

9. The Lancet Haematology Commission on sickle cell disease: key recommendations. *The Lancet Haematol*, August 2023; 10(8):e564-e567. doi: 10.1016/S2352-3026(23)00154-0. Epub 2023 Jul 11. PMID: 37451309.

10. Goldberg D.S. 'Doubt & Social Policy: The Long History of Malingering in Modern Welfare States'. *J Law Med Ethics*, 2021; 49(3):385-393. doi: 10.1017/jme.2021.58. PMID: 34665090.

11. General Medical Council. 'Preventable patient harm across health services'. 2017. https://www.gmc-uk.org/about/what-we-do-and-why/data-and-research/research-and-insight-archive/preventable-patient-harm-across-healthcare-services [accessed 15 February 2024].

12. NHS Improvement Report of the Patient Safety Initiative Group. 'Spoken communication and patient safety in the NHS'. NHS England, July 2018. https://www.england.nhs.uk/wp-content/uploads/2022/03/spoken-communication-and-patient-safety-in-the-nhs-full-report.pdf [accessed 15 February 2024].

13. Reader T.W., Gillespie A., Roberts J. 'Patient complaints in healthcare systems: a systematic review and coding taxonomy'. *BMJ Quality & Safety*, 2014;23:678-689.

14. Gawande A. *Complications: A Surgeon's Notes on an Imperfect Science*. London: Profile, 2002.

15. Cox C., Fritz Z. 'Presenting complaint: use of language that disempowers patients'. *BMJ*, 2022; 377:e066720. doi:10.1136/bmj-2021-066720.

16. Fricker M. *Epistemic Injustice: Power and the Ethics of Knowing*. Oxford: Oxford University Press, 2007.

17. Kidd I.J. and Carel H. 'Healthcare Practice, Epistemic Injustice, and Naturalism'. In Barker S. *et al*. *Harms and Wrongs in Epistemic Practice*. Cambridge: Cambridge University Press, 2018.

18. Gallagher S., Little J.M., Hooker C. 'Testimonial injustice: discounting women's voices in health care priority setting'. *Journal of Medical Ethics*, 24 April 2020. doi: 10.1136/medethics-2019-105984.

19. Dotson K. 'Tracking Epistemic Violence, Tracking Practices of Silencing'. *Hypatia* 26(2), 2011. pp236–57.

20. Sabaté E. ed. 'Adherence to Long-Term Therapies: Evidence for Action'. Geneva, Switzerland: World Health Organization, 2003.

21. Osterberg L., Blaschke T. 'Adherence to Medication'. *N Engl J Med*, 2005;353(5):487–497. doi:10.1056/NEJMra050100.

22. Martin L.R., Williams S.L., Haskard K.B., Dimatteo M.R. 'The challenge of patient adherence'. *Ther Clin Risk Manag*, September 2005;1(3):189-99. PMID: 18360559; PMCID: PMC1661624.

23. Safran D.G., Taira D.A., Rogers W.H. *et al*. 'Linking primary care performance to outcomes of care'. *J Fam Pract*, 1998; 47:213–20.

24. Graham S. 'Blaming women for being "fobbed off" shows the Government doesn't take endometriosis seriously'. *The Telegraph*, 23 October 2020. https://www.telegraph.co.uk/women/life/blaming-women-fobbed-shows-government-doesnt-take-endometriosis/ [accessed 25 February 2024].

25. Ockenden D. and Barnett E. *Woman's Hour*. BBC Radio 4, 31 March 2022.

26. Akbar A. *Consumed: A Sister's Story*. London: Sceptre, 2021.

27. Mantel H. *Giving up the Ghost: A memoir*. London: Fourth Estate, 2003.

28. Cummings L. 'Listening to Black Californians: How the Health Care System Undermines Their Pursuit of Good Health'. Califoria Health Care Foundation, 4 October 2022. https://www.chcf.org/publication/listening-black-californians-how-the-health-care-system-undermines-their-pursuit-good-health/ [accessed 15 February 2024].

29. Mills M. ' "We had such trust, we feel such fools": how shocking hospital mistakes led to our daughter's death'. *The Guardian*, 3 September 2022. https://www.theguardian.com/lifeandstyle/2022/sep/03/13-year-old-daughter-dead-in-five-weeks-hospital-mistakes [accessed 15 February 2024].

30. Birkeland S., Bismark M., Barry M.J., Möller S. 'Sociodemographic characteristics associated with a higher wish to complain about health care'. *Public Health*, 2022;210:41-47. doi:10.1016/j.puhe.2022.06.009.

31. Bismark M.M., Brennan T.A., Paterson R.J., Davis P.B., Studdert D.M.

'Relationship between complaints and quality of care in New Zealand: a descriptive analysis of complainants and non-complainants following adverse events'. *Qual Saf Health Care*, February 2006. 15(1):17-22. doi: 10.1136/qshc.2005.015743. PMID: 16456205; PMCID: PMC2563994.

32. Beard M. 'A history of laughter – from Cicero to The Simpsons'. *The Guardian*, 28 June 2014. https://www.theguardian.com/books/2014/jun/28/history-laughter-roman-jokes-mary-beard [accessed 15 February 2024].

33. NHS Improvement Report. (n 12).

2: Devalued

1. The Medical Defence Union. 'Nearly all GPs have faced a complaint during their career according to a MDU member survey'. 11 March 2021. https://www.themdu.com/press-centre/press-releases/nearly-all-gps-have-faced-a-complaint-during-their-career-mdu-member-survey [accessed 15 February 2024].

2. Chen X. 'Why We Need More Writers Practicing Medicine (and Vice Versa)'. Literary Hub, 21 March 2022. https://lithub.com/why-we-need-more-writers-practicing-medicine-and-vice-versa/ [accessed 15 February 2024].

3. Howick J., Dudko M., Feng S.N., Ahmed A.A., Alluri N., Nockels K., Winter R., Holland R. 'Why might medical student empathy change throughout medical school? A systematic review and thematic synthesis of qualitative studies'. *BMC Med Educ*, 24 April 2023. 23(1):270. doi: 10.1186/s12909-023-04165-9. PMID: 37088814; PMCID: PMC10124056.

4. Beckman H.B., Frankel R.M. 'The effect of physician behavior on the collection of data'. *Ann Intern Med*, 1984;101(5):692-696. doi:10.7326/0003-4819-101-5-692.

5. Langewitz W., Denz M., Keller A., Kiss A., Rüttimann S., Wössmer B. 'Spontaneous talking time at start of consultation in outpatient clinic: cohort study'. *BMJ*, 28 September 2002; 325(7366):682-3. doi: 10.1136/bmj.325.7366.682. PMID: 12351359; PMCID: PMC126654.

6. Beale C. 'Magical thinking and moral injury: exclusion culture in psychiatry'. *BJPsych Bull*, Feb 2022; 46(1):16-19. doi: 10.1192/bjb.2021.86. PMID: 34517935; PMCID: PMC8914811.

7. Rogers C.R., Roethlisberger F.J. 'Barriers and gateways to communication' (Reprinted from *Harvard Business Review*, July/August 1952). *Harvard Business Review*, 69, 105–111. https://hbr.org/1991/11/barriers-and-gateways-to-communication [accessed 15 February 2024].

8. Nordell J. *The End of Bias: How We Change Our Minds*. London: Granta Publications, 2021.

9. Maskell E. 'Campaigners celebrate early "amazing results" from routine HIV testing in A&E'. *Attitude*, 5 October 2022. https://www.attitude.co.uk/news/

campaigners-celebrate-early-amazing-results-from-routine-hiv-testing-in-ae%EF%BF%BC-414133/ [accessed 15 February 2024].

10. Alliance for Innovation on Maternal Health. 'Patient Safety Bundles'. https://saferbirth.org/patient-safety-bundles/ [accessed 15 February 2024].

11. Danziger S., Levav J., Avnaim-Pesso L. 'Extraneous factors in judicial decisions'. *Proc Natl Acad Sci USA*, 26 April 2011; 108(17):6889-92. doi: 10.1073/pnas.1018033108. PMID: 21482790; PMCID: PMC3084045.

12. Moorhouse A. 'Decision fatigue: less is more when making choices with patients'. *Br J Gen Pract*, 30 July 2020; 70(697):399. doi: 10.3399/bjgp20X711989. PMID: 32732206; PMCID: PMC7384807.

13. Mercer S.W., Maxwell M., Heaney D., Watt G.C. 'The consultation and relational empathy (CARE) measure: development and preliminary validation and reliability of an empathy-based consultation process measure'. *Fam Pract*, December 2004; 21(6):699-705. doi: 10.1093/fampra/cmh621. Epub 4 November 2004. PMID: 15528286.

14. Mercer S.W. 'The CARE Measure'. University of Glasgow, 2004. https://www.gla.ac.uk/media/Media_65352_smxx.pdf [accessed 15 February 2024].

15. Office for Health Improvement and Disparities. 'Patient-reported outcomes and experiences study'. gov.uk, 19 October 2020. https://www.gov.uk/guidance/patient-reported-outcomes-and-experiences-study [accessed 15 February 2024].

16. Berger J. and Mohr J. *A Fortunate Man: The Story of a Country Doctor*. New York City: Holt, Rinehart and Winston, 1967.

17. Gray D.P. 'History of the Royal College of General Practitioners – the first 40 years'. *Br J Gen Pract*, January 1992; 42(354):29-35. PMID: 1586530; PMCID: PMC1371965.

18. Morland P. and Baker R. *A Fortunate Woman: A Country Doctor's Story.* London: Picador, 2022.

19. British Medical Association. 'Pressures in general practice data analysis'. 25 January 2024. https://www.bma.org.uk/advice-and-support/nhs-delivery-and-workforce/pressures/pressures-in-general-practice-data-analysis [accessed 15 February 2024].

20. Salisbury H. 'Is transactional care enough?' *BMJ*, 28 January 2020; 368:m226. doi: 10.1136/bmj.m226. PMID: 31992553.

21. Kirmayer L.J., Groleau D., Looper K.J., Dao M.D. 'Explaining Medically Unexplained Symptoms'. *The Canadian Journal of Psychiatry*, 2004;49(10):663-672. doi:10.1177/070674370404901003.

22. Smith R. 'Death and the bogus contract between doctors and patients'. *BMJ*, 7 June 2022; 377:o1415. doi: 10.1136/bmj.o1415. PMID: 35672046.

23. Bontempo A.C. 'Patient attitudes toward clinicians' communication of diagnostic uncertainty and its impact on patient trust'. *SSM – Qualitative Research*

in Health, Volume 3, 2023, 100214, ISSN 2667-3215, https://doi.org/10.1016/j. ssmqr.2022.100214.

24. Zeldin-O'Neill, S. '"Losing sense of self": Kirsty Young opens up about illness on Desert Island Discs'. *The Guardian*, 25 December 2022. https:// www.theguardian.com/tv-and-radio/2022/dec/25/losing-sense-of-self-kirsty-young-opens-up-about-illness-on-desert-island-discs [accessed 15 February 2024].

25. Boddice R. 'The Politics of Pain'. Aeon, 3 January 2023. https://aeon.co/ essays/pain-is-not-the-purview-of-medics-what-can-historians-tell-us [accessed 15 February 2024].

26. Tomlinson J. 'Trauma and chronic pain'. A Better NHS, 1 February 2021. https://abetternhs.net/2021/02/01/trauma-and-chronic-pain/ [accessed 15 February 2024].

27. Tomlinson J. 'How Doctors respond to chronic pain', A Better NHS, 7 September 2013. https://abetternhs.net/2013/09/07/pain/ [accessed 15 February 2024].

28. Perry S. 'Out of my mind: Sarah Perry on writing under the influence of drugs'. *The Guardian*, 29 September 2018. https://www.theguardian.com/ books/2018/sep/29/high-art-writing-under-influence-drugs-sarah-perry [accessed 15 February 2024].

29. Heath I. 'The art of doing nothing'. *European Journal of General Practice*, 2012. 18:4, 242-246, doi: 10.3109/13814788.2012.733691.

30. Cassell E.J. 'The nature of suffering and the goals of medicine'. *N Engl J Med*, 18 March 1982; 306(11):639-45. doi: 10.1056/NEJM198203183061104. PMID: 7057823.

31. British Medical Association. 'Doctor patient relationship'. 26 April 2023. https://www.bma.org.uk/advice-and-support/ethics/doctor-patient-relationship/ doctor-patient-relationship [accessed 15 February 2024].

32. Ridd M., Shaw A., Lewis G., Salisbury C. 'The patient–doctor relationship: a synthesis of the qualitative literature on patients' perspectives. *Br J Gen Pract*, April 2009; 59(561):e116-33. doi: 10.3399/bjgp09X420248. PMID: 19341547; PMCID: PMC2662123.

33. Gabel L.L., Lucas J.B., Westbury R.C. 'Why do patients continue to see the same physician?' *Fam Pract Res J*, June 1993; 13(2):133-47. PMID: 8517195.

34. Huntley A., Lasserson D., Wye L., Morris R., Checkland K., England H., Salisbury C., Purdy S. 'Which features of primary care affect unscheduled secondary care use? A systematic review'. *BMJ Open*, 23 May 2014; 4(5):e004746. doi: 10.1136/bmjopen-2013-004746. PMID: 24860000; PMCID: PMC4039790.

35. Royal College of General Practitioners. 'Continuity of Care Work at RCGP'. 1 September 2021. https://www.rcgp.org.uk/blog/continuity-of-care-work-at-rcgp [accessed 10 April 2024].

36. *Psychology Today* staff. 'Transference'. *Psychology Today.* https://www.psychologytoday.com/gb/basics/transference [accessed 15 February 2024].

37. Tomlinson J. 'Emotions are Contagious'. A Better NHS and *Journal of Holistic Healthcare*, Summer 2021; 18(2). https://abetternhs.files.wordpress.com/2021/09/wp-1632927991740.pdf [accessed 15 February 2024].

38. Menzies I.E.P. 'A Case-Study in the Functioning of Social Systems as a Defence against Anxiety: A Report on a Study of the Nursing Service of a General Hospital'. *Human Relations*, 1960. 13(2), 95–121. https://doi.org/10.1177/001872676001300201.

39. Launer J. 'Conversations Inviting Change'. *Postgraduate Medical Journal*, 2008; 84:4-5 https://doi.org/10.1136/pgmj.2007.067009.

40. Shale S. 'Moral injury and the COVID-19 pandemic: reframing what it is, who it affects and how care leaders can manage it'. *BMJ Leader*, 2020; 4:224-227 https://doi.org/10.1136/leader-2020-000295.

41. Hodkinson A., Zhou A., Johnson J., Geraghty K., Riley R., Zhou A. *et al.* 'Associations of physician burnout with career engagement and quality of patient care: systematic review and meta-analysis'. *BMJ*, 2022; 378:e070442 doi:10.1136/bmj-2022-070442.

42. Beck R.S., Daughtridge R., Sloane P.D. 'Physician–patient communication in the primary care office: a systematic review'. *J Am Board Fam Pract*, 2002;15(1):25-38.

43. Mannix K. *Listen: How to Find the Words for Tender Conversations.* London: William Collins, 2021.

44. NHS England. 'What is revalidation?'. https://www.england.nhs.uk/professional-standards/medical-revalidation/about-us/what-is-revalidation/ [accessed 10 April 2024].

45. General Medical Council. 'Good Medical Practice'. 2024. https://www.gmc-uk.org/professional-standards/professional-standards-for-doctors/good-medical-practice [accessed 10 April 2024].

46. Mueller L. 'Monet Refuses the Operation'. Poetry Foundation, 1996. https://www.poetryfoundation.org/poems/52577/monet-refuses-the-operation-56d231289e6db [accessed 15 February 2024].

3: Excluded

1. Clance P.R., Imes S.A. 'The Impostor Phenomenon in High Achieving Women: Dynamics and Therapeutic Intervention'. *Psychotherapy: Theory, Research and Practice*, 1978. 15 (3): 241–247. https://doi.org/10.1037/h0086006.

2. Bravata D.M., Watts S.A., Keefer A.L. *et al.* 'Prevalence, Predictors, and Treatment of Impostor Syndrome: a Systematic Review'. *J Gen Intern Med*, 2020;35(4):1252-1275. doi:10.1007/s11606-019-05364-1.

3. Fricker M. *Epistemic Injustice: Power and the Ethics of Knowing*. Oxford: Oxford University Press, 2007.

4. Sieghart M.A. *The Authority Gap: Why women are still taken less seriously than men and what we can do about it*. London: Doubleday, 2021.

5. Gallagher S., Little J.M., Hooker C. 'Testimonial injustice: discounting women's voices in health care priority setting'. *J Med Ethics*, 2021;47(11):744-747. doi:10.1136/medethics-2019-105984.

6. Slawson N. ' "Women have been woefully neglected": does medical science have a gender problem?'. *The Guardian*, 18 November 2019. https://www.the-guardian.com/education/2019/dec/18/women-have-been-woefully-neglected-does-medical-science-have-a-gender-problem [accessed 19 February 2024].

7. Morehouse K.N., Kurdi B., Hakim E., Banaji M.R. 'When a stereotype dumbfounds: Probing the nature of the surgeon = male belief'. *Current Research in Ecological and Social Psychology*, 2022, 3, 100044 ISSN 2666-6227.

8. BBC History. 'Elizabeth Garrett Anderson (1836–1917)'. 2014. https://www.bbc.co.uk/history/historic_figures/garrett_anderson_elizabeth.shtml [accessed 19 February 2024].

9. Medical Schools Council. 'Selection Alliance 2018 Report'. 27 November 2018. https://www.medschools.ac.uk/our-work/publications?Category=2318 [accessed 10 April 2024].

10. Newman T.H., Parry M.G., Zakeri R. *et al.* 'Gender diversity in UK surgical specialties: a national observational study'. *BMJ Open*, 2022;12:e055516. doi: 10.1136/bmjopen-2021-055516.

11. The Royal College of Surgeons. 'How We Got Here: The Kennedy Report'. 2021. https://diversity.rcseng.ac.uk/how-we-got-here/ [accessed 10 April 2024].

12. Trueland J. 'Sexism and Surgery'. BMA.org.uk, 16 February 2022. https://www.bma.org.uk/news-and-opinion/sexism-and-surgery [accessed 19 February 2024].

13. Newlands C., Jackson P., Cuming T. 'Breaking the silence: addressing sexual misconduct in healthcare'. Working Party on Sexual Misconduct in Surgery (WPSMS). WPSMS.org.uk, September 2023. https://www.wpsms.org.uk/ [accessed 19 February 2024].

14. Hopkins C. @SnotSurgeon. Twitter.com, 10 February 2021. https://twitter.com/SnotSurgeon/status/1359432716303929352?s=20&t=KpcWvk6nITdsFtczRyvlzA [accessed 19 February 2024].

15. Hopkins C. @SnotSurgeon. Twitter.com, 7 October 2023. https://twitter.com/SnotSurgeon/status/1710597435494400307?s=20 [accessed 19 February 2024].

16. *BBC Question Time*. Mentorn Media. BBC 1, 4 June 2020.

17. Deihl A., Dzubinski L. 'We need to stop "untitling" and "uncredentialing" professional women'. *Fast Company*, 22 January 2021. https://www.fastcompany.com/90596628/we-need-to-stop-untitling-and-uncredentialing-professional-women [accessed 19 February 2024].

18. Files J.A., Mayer A.P., Ko M.G. *et al.* 'Speaker Introductions at Internal Medicine Grand Rounds: Forms of Address Reveal Gender Bias'. *J Women's Health (Larchmt)*, 2017;26(5):413-419. doi:10.1089/jwh.2016.6044.

19. British Medical Association. 'Sexism in Medicine Survey Report'. August 2021. https://www.bma.org.uk/media/4488/sexism-in-medicine-bma-report-august-2021.pdf [accessed 19 February 2024].

20. Surviving in Scrubs. 'Your Stories'. https://survivinginscrubsorg.wordpress.com/your-stories/ [accessed 19 February 2024].

21. Department of Health and Social Care. 'Mend the Gap: The Independent Review into Gender Pay Gaps in Medicine in England'. gov.uk, December 2020. https://assets.publishing.service.gov.uk/government/uploads/system/uploads/attachment_data/file/944246/Gender_pay_gap_in_medicine_review.pdf [accessed 22 March 2024].

22. Puwar N. *Space Invaders: Race, Gender and Bodies Out of Place.* New York: Berg Publishers, 2004.

23. Begum S. *et al.* 'Broken Ladders: The myth of meritocracy for women of colour in the workplace'. The Fawcett Society and The Runnymede Trust, 2022. https://www.runnymedetrust.org//publications/broken-ladders [accessed 19 February 2024].

24. Pery S., Doytch G., and Kluger A.N. 'Management and leadership', in Worthington D.L. and Bodie G.D. Hoboken (eds.). *The Handbook of Listening.* New Jersey: Wiley, 2020, pp163–179.

25. Kriz T.D., Kluger A.N., Lyddy C.J. 'Feeling Heard: Experiences of Listening (or Not) at Work'. *Front Psychol*, 26 July 2021. 2021;12:659087. doi: 10.3389/fpsyg.2021.659087.

26. Imtiaz-Umer S. and Frain J. *ABC of Equality, Diversity and Inclusion in Healthcare.* Hoboken, New Jersey: Wiley-Blackwell, 2023.

27. Friedman S., Laurison D. *The Class Ceiling: Why it Pays to Be Privileged.* Bristol: Policy Press, 2020.

28. Haque E., Spencer A., Alldridge L. 'Developing a UK widening participation forum'. *Clin Teach*, October 2021;18(5):482-484. https://doi.org/10.1111/tct.13357.

29. Dawson J. 'Links between NHS Staff Experience and Patient Satisfaction: Analysis of surveys from 2014 and 2015'. NHS England, 2018. https://www.england.nhs.uk/wp-content/uploads/2018/02/links-between-nhs-staff-experience-and-patient-satisfaction-1.pdf [accessed 22 March].

30. Alsan M., Garrick O., Graziani G. 'Does Diversity Matter for Health?' Experimental Evidence from Oakland (June 2018). NBER Working Paper No. w24787. https://ssrn.com/abstract=3210441 [accessed 19 February 2024].

31. Snyder J.E., Upton R.D., Hassett T.C., Lee H., Nouri Z., Dill M. 'Black Representation in the Primary Care Physician Workforce and Its Association

with Population Life Expectancy and Mortality Rates in the US'. *JAMA Netw Open*, 3 April 2023;6(4):e236687. doi: 10.1001/jamanetworkopen.2023.6687. PMID: 37058307; PMCID: PMC10105312.

32. Malhotra J., Rotter D., Tsui J., Llanos A.A.M., Balasubramanian B.A., Demissie K. 'Impact of Patient-Provider Race, Ethnicity, and Gender Concordance on Cancer Screening: Findings from Medical Expenditure Panel Survey'. *Cancer Epidemiol Biomarkers Prev*, 2017;26(12):1804-1811. doi: 10.1158/1055-9965.EPI-17-0660.

33. LaVeist T.A., Nuru-Jeter A., Jones K.E. 'The association of doctor–patient race concordance with health services utilization'. *J Public Health Policy*, 2003;24(3-4):312-323 PMID: 15015865.

34. Greenwood B.N., Hardeman R.R., Huang L., Sojourner A. 'Physician–patient racial concordance and disparities in birthing mortality for newborns'. *Proc Natl Acad Sci USA*, 2020;117(35):21194-21200. doi: 10.1073/pnas.1913405117.

35. Street Jr. R.L., O'Malley K.J., Cooper L.A., Haidet P. 'Understanding concordance in patient–physician relationships: personal and ethnic dimensions of shared identity'. *Ann Fam Med*, 2008;6(3):198–205. doi: 10.1370/afm.821.

36. Sabaté E. ed. 'Adherence to Long-Term Therapies: Evidence for Action'. Geneva, Switzerland: World Health Organization, 2003.

37. Simpson J.M., Esmail A., Kalra V.S., Snow S.J. 'Writing migrants back into NHS history: addressing a "collective amnesia" and its policy implications'. *J R Soc Med*, 2010 Oct;103(10):392-6. doi: 10.1258/jrsm.2010.100222. Epub 9 September 2010. PMID: 20829323; PMCID: PMC2951177.

38. Naqvi H., Williams R.D. 2nd, Chinembiri O., Rodger S. 'Workforce and workplace racism in health systems: organisations are diverse but not inclusive'. *The Lancet*, 10 December 2022. 10;400(10368):2023-2026. doi: 10.1016/S0140-6736(22)02395-9. PMID: 36502831; PMCID: PMC9731575.

39. British Medical Association. 'Racism in Medicine Survey Report'. June 2022. https://www.bma.org.uk/media/5746/bma-racism-in-medicine-survey-report-15-june-2022.pdf [accessed 19 February 2024].

40. Royal College of Nursing. 'Employment Survey Report 2021: Workforce diversity and employment experiences'. 8 June 2022. https://www.rcn.org.uk/professional-development/publications/Employment-Survey-Report-2021-uk-pub-010-216 [accessed 19 February 2024].

41. NHS Workforce Race Equality Standard. '2021 Data Analysis Report for NHS Trusts'. NHS England, March 2022. https://www.england.nhs.uk/wp-content/uploads/2022/04/Workforce-Race-Equality-Standard-report-2021-.pdf [accessed 19 February 2024].

42. Woodhead C., Stoll N., Harwood H., TIDES Study Team, Alexis O., Hatch S.L. '"They created a team of almost entirely the people who work and are like them": A qualitative study of organisational culture and racialised

inequalities among healthcare staff'. *Sociol Health Illn*, 2022;44(2):267-289. doi:10.1111/1467-9566.13414.

43. Dill J., Duffy M. 'Structural Racism and Black Women's Employment In The US Health Care Sector'. *Health Aff (Millwood)*, February 2022;41(2):265-272. doi: 10.1377/hlthaff.2021.01400. PMID: 35130061; PMCID: PMC9281878.

44. Ly D.P., Seabury S.A., Jena A.B. 'Differences in incomes of physicians in the United States by race and sex: observational study'. *BMJ*, 7 June 2016;353:i2923. doi: 10.1136/bmj.i2923. PMID: 27268490; PMCID: PMC4897176.

45. Corrigan C. 'Disabled doctors deserve to be heard'. BMA.org, 4 July 2023. https://www.bma.org.uk/news-and-opinion/disabled-doctors-deserve-to-be-heard [accessed 19 February 2024].

46. Imtiaz-Umer S. *et al.* (n 26).

47. Malik A., Qureshi H., Abdul-Razakq H. *et al.* ' "I decided not to go into surgery due to dress code": a cross-sectional study within the UK investigating experiences of female Muslim medical health professionals on bare below the elbows (BBE) policy and wearing headscarves (hijabs) in theatre'. *BMJ Open*, 2019;9:e019954. doi: 10.1136/bmjopen-2017-019954.

48. Kline R., Lewis D. 'The price of fear: Estimating the financial cost of bullying and harassment to the NHS in England'. *Public Money Manag*, 2019;39:166-74. doi:10.1080/09540962.2018.1535044.

49. Hemmings N., Buckingham H., Oung C., Palmer W. 'Attracting and retaining a diverse NHS workforce'. Research Report, Nuffield Trust, 8 November 2021. https://www.nuffieldtrust.org.uk/research/attracting-supporting-and-retaining-a-diverse-nhs-workforce [accessed 19 February 2024].

50. Gopal D.P., Chetty U., O'Donnell P., Gajria C., Blackadder-Weinstein J. 'Implicit bias in healthcare: clinical practice, research and decision making'. *Future Healthc J*, 2021;8(1):40-48. doi:10.7861/fhj.2020-0233.

51. The Active Bystander. 'The Active Bystander Training Company'. https://www.activebystander.co.uk/ [accessed 19 February 2024].

52. Eckert M. 'Civil rights leader Angela Davis speaks at Bovard'. *Daily Trojan*, 23 February 2015. https://dailytrojan.com/2015/02/23/civil-rights-leader-angela-davis-speaks-at-bovard/ [accessed 19 February 2024].

53. Dhairyawan R. 'Evaluating Values'. *BMJ Leader*, 15 June 2020. https://blogs.bmj.com/bmjleader/2020/06/15/evaluating-values-by-rageshri-dhairyawan/ [accessed 19 February 2024].

4: Missing

1. Dhairyawan R. 'Work in Progress' in Brown K. ed. *No One Talks About This Stuff*. London: Unbound, 2024.

2. Ghai V., Jan H., Shakir F., Haines P., Kent A. 'Diagnostic delay for superficial

and deep endometriosis in the United Kingdom'. *J Obstet Gynaecol*, January 2020;40(1):83-89. doi: 10.1080/01443615.2019.1603217. Epub 22 July 2019. PMID: 31328629.

3. World Health Organization. 'Endometriosis Factsheet'. 24 March 2023. https://www.who.int/news-room/fact-sheets/detail/endometriosis [accessed 19 February 2024].

4. Mousa M., Al-Jefout M., Alsafar H., Becker C.M., Zondervan K.T., Rahmioglu N. 'Impact of Endometriosis in Women of Arab Ancestry on: Health-Related Quality of Life, Work Productivity, and Diagnostic Delay'. *Front Glob Womens Health*, 14 September 2021;2:708410. doi: 10.3389/fgwh.2021.708410. PMID: 34816238; PMCID: PMC8593935.

5. Armour M., Sinclair J., Ng C.H.M., Hyman M.S., Lawson K., Smith C.A., Abbott J. 'Endometriosis and chronic pelvic pain have similar impact on women, but time to diagnosis is decreasing: an Australian survey'. *Sci Rep*, 1 October 2020;10(1):16253. doi: 10.1038/s41598-020-73389-2. PMID: 33004965; PMCID: PMC7529759.

6. Bougie O., Yap M.I., Sikora L., Flaxman T., Singh S. 'Influence of race/ethnicity on prevalence and presentation of endometriosis: a systematic review and meta-analysis'. *BJOG*, August 2019;126(9):1104-1115. doi: 10.1111/1471-0528.15692. Epub 29 April 2019. PMID: 30908874.

7. Dawood M.Y. 'Dysmenorrhea'. *J Reprod Med*, March 1985;30(3):154-67. PMID: 3158737.

8. Virdi J. 'Painful Realities' series, Wellcome Collection Stories, 2019. https://wellcomecollection.org/series/XTg5pRAAACUAP5U5 [accessed 19 February 2024].

9. Meigs J.V. 'Endometriosis; etiologic role of marriage age and parity; conservative treatment'. *Obstet Gynecol*, July 1953;2(1):46-53. PMID: 13073079.

10. Farland L.V., Horne A.W. 'Disparity in endometriosis diagnoses between racial/ethnic groups'. *BJOG*, August 2019;126(9):1115-1116. doi: 10.1111/1471-0528.15805. Epub 21 May 2019. PMID: 31033134; PMCID: PMC6767495:

11. Gross R.E. *Vagina Obscura: An Anatomical Voyage*. New York: WW Norton and Co, 2022.

12. Graham S. 'My endometriosis was treated like a character flaw rather than a medical condition'. *I News*, 5 January 2023. https://inews.co.uk/inews-lifestyle/treated-endometriosis-character-flaw-medical-condition-2063264 [accessed 19 February 2024].

13. Hintz E.A. ' "It's All in Your Head": A Meta-Synthesis of Qualitative Research About Disenfranchising Talk Experienced by Female Patients with Chronic Overlapping Pain Conditions'. *Health Commun*, 12 June 2022:1-15. doi: 10.1080/10410236.2022.2081046. PMID: 35694781.

14. Dennett K., Johnston H. 'Woman, 23, who has to use a wheelchair and is

unable to go to the bathroom alone due to endometriosis says she "can't" have a hysterectomy on the NHS because she's "too young and hasn't had children"'. *The Daily Mail*, 15 April 2021. https://www.dailymail.co.uk/femail/article-9474415/Endometriosis-Woman-claims-refused-hysterectomy-age.html [accessed 19 February 2024].

15. Ellis K., Munro D., Clarke J. 'Endometriosis Is Undervalued: A Call to Action'. *Front Glob Women's Health*, 10 May 2022;3:902371. doi: 10.3389/fgwh.2022.902371. PMID: 35620300; PMCID: PMC9127440.

16. Mirin A.A. 'Gender Disparity in the Funding of Diseases by the U.S. National Institutes of Health'. *J Women's Health (Larchmt)*, July 2021;30(7):956-963. doi: 10.1089/jwh.2020.8682. Epub 27 Nov 2020. PMID: 33232627; PMCID: PMC8290307.

17. Slawson N. '"Women have been woefully neglected": does medical science have a gender problem?'. *The Guardian*, 18 November 2019. https://www.the-guardian.com/education/2019/dec/18/women-have-been-woefully-neglected-does-medical-science-have-a-gender-problem [accessed 19 February 2024].

18. Gross R.E. (n 11).

19. Wahlquist C. 'The sole function of the clitoris is female orgasm. Is that why it's ignored by medical science?'. *The Guardian*, 31 October 2020. https://www.theguardian.com/lifeandstyle/2020/nov/01/the-sole-function-of-the-clitoris-is-female-orgasm-is-that-why-its-ignored-by-medical-science [accessed 19 February 2024].

20. Irving R. 'Ailsa Irving obituary'. *The Guardian*, 13 December 2022. https://www.theguardian.com/society/2022/dec/13/ailsa-irving-obituary [accessed 19 February 2024].

21. Endometriosis.org. 'Recognising endometriosis advocates: Ailsa Irving'. 2024. https://endometriosis.org/news/support-awareness/recognising-endometriosis-advocates-ailsa-irving/ [accessed 19 February 2024].

22. Endometriosis UK. 'About Us'. Endometriosis UK Annual Report 2022. https://www.endometriosis-uk.org/about-us [accessed 19 February 2024].

23. Adelaine, A. *et al.* 'Knowledge Is Power – An Open Letter To UKRI'. Research Professional News, 17 August 2020. https://www.researchprofessionalnews.com/rr-news-uk-views-of-the-uk-2020-8-knowledge-is-power-an-open-letter-to-ukri/ [accessed 19 February 2024].

24. UK Research and Innovation. 'Diversity data for funding applicants and awardees 2020-21'. 1 December 2022. https://www.ukri.org/publications/diversity-data-for-funding-applicants-and-awardees-2020-21/ [accessed 19 February 2024].

25. National Institute for Health and Care Research. 'Diversity Data Report 2020/21'. December 2021. https://www.nihr.ac.uk/documents/diversity-data-report-202021/29410 [accessed 19 February 2024].

26. Dandar V., Lautenberger D. 'Exploring Faculty Salary Equity at U.S. Medical Schools by Gender and Race/Ethnicity'. Association of American Medical Colleges, October 2021. https://store.aamc.org/downloadable/download/sample/sample_id/453/ [accessed 19 February 2024].

27. Hoppe T.A., Litovitz A., Willis K.A., Meseroll R.D., Perkins M.J. *et al.* 'Topic choice contributes to the lower rate of NIH awards to African-American/black scientists'. *Science Advances*, 9 October 2019. doi: 10.1126/sciadv.aaw7238.

28. Salway S., Holman D., Lee C., McGowan V., Ben-Shlomo Y., Saxena S *et al.* 'Transforming the health system for the UK's multiethnic population', *BMJ*, 2020; 368:m268 doi: https://doi.org/10.1136/bmj.m268.

29. Liu F., Rahwan T., AlShebli B. 'Non-White scientists appear on fewer editorial boards, spend more time under review, and receive fewer citations'. *Proc Natl Acad Sci USA*, 28 March 2023;120(13):e2215324120. doi: 10.1073/pnas.2215324120. Epub 20 Mar 2023. PMID: 36940343.

30. Gibney E. 'How UK science is failing Black researchers – in nine stark charts'. *Nature*, 14 December 2022. https://www.nature.com/immersive/d41586-022-04386-w/index.html [accessed 19 February 2024].

31. Ibid.

32. Dandar V. (n 26).

33. Blackstock U. 'Why Black doctors like me are leaving faculty positions in academic medical centers'. Stat News, 16 January 2020. https://www.statnews.com/2020/01/16/black-doctors-leaving-faculty-positions-academic-medical-centers/ [accessed 19 February 2024].

34. TigerinSTEMM. 'Barriers to accessing funding'. 2022. https://www.tigerin-stemm.org/resources/barriers-to-funding [accessed 19 February 2024].

35. TigerinSTEMM. 'Barriers LGBTQI+ People Face in the Research Funding Processes'. OSF Preprints, 16 November 2019. doi:10.31219/osf.io/dnhv8.

36. TigerinSTEMM. (n 34).

37. TigerinSTEMM. 'Accessibility in STEM: Barriers Facing Disabled Individuals in Research Funding Processes'. OSF Preprints, 2 December 2019. doi:10.31219/osf.io/uzsdk.

38. Gibney E. (n 30).

39. Gladstone J. *et al.* 'Equity and Inclusivity in Research Funding: Barriers and Delivering Change'. University of Oxford, 2022. https://researchsupport.admin.ox.ac.uk/files/equityandinclusivityinresearchfundingpdf [accessed 19 February 2024].

40. Dhairyawan R., Tariq S., Scourse R., Coyne K.M. 'Intimate partner violence in women living with HIV attending an inner-city clinic in the UK: prevalence and associated factors'. *HIV Med*, May 2013;14(5):303-10. doi: 10.1111/hiv.12009. Epub 6 Dec 2012. PMID: 23217089.

41. NHS Health Research Authority. 'Research Ethics Service and Research Ethics

Committees'. https://www.hra.nhs.uk/about-us/committees-and-services/res-and-recs/ [accessed 19 February 2024].

42. World Health Organization. 'Consolidated guideline on sexual and reproductive health and rights of women living with HIV – Guideline'. 16 May 2019. https://www.who.int/publications/i/item/9789241549998 [accessed 19 February 2024].

43. Dotson K. 'Conceptualizing Epistemic Oppression'. *Social Epistemology*, 16 January 2014;28(2):115–138. doi: 10.1080/02691728.2013.782585.

44. *The Lancet* Series. 'The Lancet Series on racism, xenophobia, discrimination, and health'. *The Lancet*, 8 December 2022. https://www.thelancet.com/series/racism-xenophobia-discrimination-health [accessed 19 February 2024].

45. The Wellcome Trust. 'The History of Wellcome'. https://wellcome.org/who-we-are/history-wellcome [accessed 19 February 2024].

46. The Wellcome Trust. 'Press Release: Our commitment to tackling racism at Wellcome'. 17 June 2020. https://wellcome.org/press-release/our-commitment-tackling-racism-wellcome [accessed 19 February 2024].

47. The Wellcome Trust. 'Report Summary: Grant funding data 2019 to 2020'. 26 March 2021. https://wellcome.org/reports/grant-funding-data-2019-2020 [accessed 19 February 2024].

48. The Wellcome Trust. 'Diversity, equity and inclusion strategy'. https://wellcome.org/what-we-do/diversity-and-inclusion/strategy [accessed 19 February 2024].

49. The Wellcome Trust. 'Press Release: "Insufficient progress" on anti-racism at Wellcome, evaluation finds'. 10 August 2022. https://wellcome.org/news/insufficient-progress-anti-racism-wellcome-evaluation-finds [accessed 19 February 2024].

50. Ibid.

51. Ibid.

52. Ahmed S. *Complaint!* Durham: Duke University Press, 2021.

53. Subramaniam B. and Wyer M. 'Assimilating the "Culture of No Culture" in Science: Feminist Interventions in (De)Mentoring Graduate Women'. *Feminist Teacher*, 1998, 12(1): pp12–28.

54. The Wellcome Trust. 'Statement on the closure of our Medicine Man gallery'. 28 November 2022. https://wellcomecollection.org/pages/Y4TdMBAAACMApBI4 [accessed 19 February 2024].

55. Koplan J.P., Bond T.C., Merson M.H., Reddy K.S., Rodriguez M.H., Sewankambo N.K. *et al.* 'Towards a common definition of global health'. *The Lancet*, 2009;373:1993–5. doi: 10.1016/S0140-6736(09)60332-9.

56. Pai M. 'Disrupting Global Health: From Allyship to Collective Liberation'. *Forbes*, 15 March 2022. https://www.forbes.com/sites/madhukarpai/2022/03/15/disrupting-global-health-from-allyship-to-collective-liberation/?sh=c2248304e623 [accessed 19 February 2024].

57. Kunitz S.J. *Disease and Social Diversity: The European Impact on the Health of Non-Europeans*. New York: Oxford University Press, 1994.

58. Global Health 50/50. 'The Global Health 50/50 Report 2020: Power, Privilege and Priorities'. London, 2020. https://globalhealth5050.org/wp-content/uploads/2020/03/Power-Privilege-and-Priorities-2020-Global-Health-5050-Report.pdf [accessed 19 February 2024].

59. Packard R.M. *A History of Global Health: Interventions Into the Lives of Other Peoples*. Baltimore: Johns Hopkins University Press, 2016.

60. World Health Organization. 'Traditional medicine has a long history of contributing to conventional medicine and continues to hold promise'. 10 August 2023. https://www.who.int/news-room/feature-stories/detail/traditional-medicine-has-a-long-history-of-contributing-to-conventional-medicine-and-continues-to-hold-promise [accessed 19 February 2024].

61. Norton K. 'How African Indigenous knowledge helped shape modern medicine'. Nova, PBS.org, 30 March 2022. https://www.pbs.org/wgbh/nova/article/smallpox-epidemic-boston-onesimus-african-indigenous/ [accessed 19 February 2024].

62. Iacobelli T. 'The Rockefeller Foundation's 20th-Century Global Fight Against Disease: The Start of Something Big'. RE:source, Rockefeller Archive Centre, 6 January 2022. https://resource.rockarch.org/story/the-rockefeller-foundations-20th-century-global-fight-against-disease/ [accessed 19 February 2024].

63. Packard R.M. (n 59).

64. Ibid.

65. Patel R. and Marya R. *Inflamed: Deep Medicine and the Anatomy of Injustice*. London: Allen Lane, 2021.

66. Dotson K. 'Tracking Epistemic Violence, Tracking Practices of Silencing'. *Hypatia*, 2011; 26(2): 236–57. https://doi.org/10.1111/j.1527-2001.2011.01177.x.

67. World Health Organization. 'Neglected tropical diseases Q&A'. January 2024. https://www.who.int/news-room/questions-and-answers/item/neglected-tropical-diseases [accessed 19 February 2024].

68. 'The Global Health 50/50 Report 2020' (n 58).

69. Ibid.

70. Bhakuni H., Abimbola S. 'Epistemic injustice in academic global health'. *The Lancet Glob Health*, 2021;9(10):e1465-e1470. doi:10.1016/S2214-109X(21)00301-6.

71. Waruru M. 'Renowned journal rejects papers that exclude African researchers'. University World News, 3 June 2022. https://www.universityworldnews.com/post.php?story=20220603115640789 [accessed 19 February 2024].

72. Marginson S. and Xu X. 'Moving beyond centre-periphery science: Towards an ecology of knowledge'. Working paper no. 63, Centre for Global Higher Education, April 2021. https://www.researchcghe.org/publications/

working-paper/moving-beyond-centre-periphery-science-towards-an-ecology-of-knowledge/ [accessed 19 February 2024].

73. Floyd L., Stauss M., Woywodt A. 'Is open access a misnomer?' *The Lancet*, 26 March 2022;399(10331):1226. doi: 10.1016/S0140-6736(22)00107-6. PMID: 35339224.

74. Byanyima W. @Winnie_Byanyima. Twitter.com, 26 July 2022. https://twitter.com/Winnie_Byanyima/status/1551888877316710400 [accessed 19 February 2024].

75. Johnson T. @tianjohnson. Twitter.com, 26 July 2022. https://twitter.com/tianjohnson/status/1551974562245509121 [accessed 19 February 2024].

76. International AIDS Society. 'IAS announces global rotation of all its conferences'. 14 February 2023. https://www.iasociety.org/news/ias-announces-global-rotation-all-its-conferences [accessed 19 February 2024].

77. Tuhiwai Smith L. *Decolonizing Methodologies: Research and Indigenous Peoples*. London: Zed Books, 2021 (3rd edition).

78. Prasad A. 'Thirusha Naidu: Shifting Power and Changing Practice'. *The Lancet*, 2022; 400 (10368). https://doi.org/10.1016/S0140-6736(22)02497-7.

79. Smeeth L. and Kyobutungi C. 'Reclaiming Global Health'. *The Lancet*, February 2023. 2023; 401 (10377). https://doi.org/10.1016/S0140-6736(23)00327-6.

80. Kumar M. *et al.* 'What should equity in global health research look like?'. *The Lancet*, 18 May 2022. https://www.thelancet.com/journals/lancet/article/PIIS0140-6736(22)00888-1/fulltext#%20 [accessed 19 February 2024].

81. Hirsch L.A. 'Is it possible to decolonise global health institutions?' *The Lancet*, 16 January 2021;397(10270):189-190. doi: 10.1016/S0140-6736(20)32763-X. PMID: 33453772.

5: Objective

1. NHS England. 'Shared decision-making'. https://www.england.nhs.uk/personalisedcare/shared-decision-making/ [accessed 20 February 2024].

2. Chowdhury S.R., Chandra Das D., Sunna T.C., Beyene J., Hossain A. 'Global and regional prevalence of multimorbidity in the adult population in community settings: a systematic review and meta-analysis'. *EClinicalMedicine*, 16 February 2023;57:101860. doi: 10.1016/j.eclinm.2023.101860. PMID: 36864977; PMCID: PMC9971315.

3. Ipsos. 'Doctors become the world's most trusted profession'. 12 October 2021. https://www.ipsos.com/en-uk/doctors-become-worlds-most-trusted-profession [accessed 20 February 2024].

4. Definition of 'objective' in *Collins COBUILD Advanced Learner's Dictionary*. London: HarperCollins Publishers, 2024. https://www.collinsdictionary.com/dictionary/english/objective [accessed 20 February 2024].

5. Lantz P.M., Goldberg D.S., Gollust S.E. 'The Perils of Medicalization for Population Health and Health Equity'. *Milbank Q*, April 2023;101(S1):61-82. doi: 10.1111/1468-0009.12619. PMID: 37096631; PMCID: PMC10126964.

6. General Medical Council. 'Our history'. https://www.gmc-uk.org/about/who-we-are/our-history [accessed 20 February 2024].

7. Semmelweis I. *Etiology, Concept and Prophylaxis of Childbed Fever*. Trans. Codell Carter K. Wisconsin: University of Wisconsin Press, 1983.

8. Best M., Neuhauser D. 'Ignaz Semmelweis and the birth of infection control'. *BMJ Quality & Safety*, 2004;13:233-234. https://doi.org/10.1136/qshc.2004.010918.

9. Cleghorn E. 'Invisible mothers & invisible monster: The journey to modern maternity medicine'. Programme from *Dr Semmelweiss* play, Harold Pinter Theatre, London, 2023.

10. Webb W.M. 'Rationalism, Empiricism, and Evidence-Based Medicine: A Call for a New Galenic Synthesis'. *Medicines*, 2018; 5(2):40. https://doi.org/10.3390/medicines5020040.

11. Our Bodies Ourselves Today. 'The History & Legacy of Our Bodies Ourselves'. https://www.ourbodiesourselves.org/about-us/our-history/ [accessed 20 February 2024].

12. Library of Congress. 'Books That Shaped America 1950 to 2000'. https://www.loc.gov/exhibits/books-that-shaped-america/1950-to-2000.html [accessed 20 February 2024].

13. Boston Women's Health Book Collective. *Our Bodies, Ourselves: A New Edition for a New Era*. New York: Simon and Schuster, 2011.

14. Dickersin K., Straus S.E., Bero L.A. 'Evidence based medicine: increasing, not dictating, choice', *BMJ*, 2007; 334 :s10 doi:10.1136/bmj.39062.639444.94.

15. Sheridan D.J., Julian D.G. 'Achievements and Limitations of Evidence-Based Medicine'. *J Am Coll Cardiol*, 12 July 2016;68(2):204-13. doi: 10.1016/j.jacc.2016.03.600. PMID: 27386775.

16. Burns P.B., Rohrich R.J., Chung K.C. 'The levels of evidence and their role in evidence-based medicine'. *Plast Reconstr Surg*, July 2011;128(1):305-310. doi: 10.1097/PRS.0b013e318219c171. PMID: 21701348; PMCID: PMC3124652.

17. National Information Center on Health Services Research and Health Care Technology (NICHSR). 'Introduction to Health Services Research: A Self-Study Course'. U.S. National Library of Medicine, November 2007. http://wayback.archive-it.org/org-350/20180515160859/https://www.nlm.nih.gov/nichsr/ihcm/06studies/studies03.html [accessed 20 February 2024].

18. Lehman R., Mehta R. *Richard Lehman on Evidence Based Medicine* podcast, 2022. https://podcasts.apple.com/gb/podcast/richard-lehman-on-evidence-based-medicine/id1636203466 [accessed 26 March 2024].

19. Cochrane. 'About Us'. https://www.cochrane.org/about-us [accessed 20 February 2024].

20. British Medical Journal. 'How to Read A Paper'. https://www.bmj.com/about-bmj/resources-readers/publications/how-read-paper [accessed 20 February 2024].

21. Sense About Science. 'Evidence Based Medicine Matters: Example of where EBM has benefitted patients'. Testing Treatments International, 2013. https://en.testingtreatments.org/evidence-based-medicine-matters/ [accessed 20 February 2024].

22. Wikipedia. 'Patrick Bouvier Kennedy'. February 2024. https://en.wikipedia.org/wiki/Patrick_Bouvier_Kennedy [accessed 20 February 2024].

23. AllTrials. 'What does all trials registered and reported mean?'. September 2013. https://www.alltrials.net/find-out-more/all-trials/ [accessed 20 February 2024].

24. Goldacre B. *Bad Pharma*. London: Fourth Estate, 2012.

25. Goldberg D.S. 'Pain, objectivity and history: understanding pain stigma'. *Med Humanit*, December 2017;43(4):238-243. doi: 10.1136/medhum-2016-011133. Epub 21 February 2017. PMID: 28228477.

26. Album D., Johannessen L.E.F., Rasmussen E.B. 'Stability and change in disease prestige: A comparative analysis of three surveys spanning a quarter of a century'. *Soc Sci Med*, 2017;180:45-51. doi:10.1016/j.socscimed.2017.03.020.

27. Bernstein J. 'Not the Last Word: Fibromyalgia is Real'. *Clin Orthop Relat Res*, February 2016;474(2):304-9. doi: 10.1007/s11999-015-4670-6. Epub 16 December 2015. PMID: 26676117; PMCID: PMC4709307.

28. Heggen K.M., Berg H. 'Epistemic injustice in the age of evidence-based practice: The case of fibromyalgia'. *Humanit Soc Sci Commun*, 2021; 8, 235. https://doi.org/10.1057/s41599-021-00918-3.

29. Clauw D.J., D'Arcy Y., Gebke K., Semel D., Pauer L., Jones K.D. 'Normalizing fibromyalgia as a chronic illness'. *Postgrad Med*, January 2018;130(1):9-18. doi: 10.1080/00325481.2018.1411743. Epub 19 December 2017. PMID: 29256764.

30. Farooq H.Z., Apea V., Kasadha B. *et al.* 'Study protocol: the ILANA study – exploring optimal implementation strategies for long-acting antiretroviral therapy to ensure equity in clinical care and policy for women, racially minoritized people and older people living with HIV in the UK – a qualitative multiphase longitudinal study design'. *BMJ Open*, 2023;13:e070666. doi: 10.1136/bmjopen-2022-070666.

31. Nooney J., Thor S., de Vries C., Clements J., Sahin L., Hua W., Everett D., Zaccaria C., Ball R., Saint-Raymond A., Yao L., Raine J., Kweder S. 'Assuring Access to Safe Medicines in Pregnancy and Breastfeeding'. *Clin Pharmacol Ther*, October 2021;110(4):941-945. doi: 10.1002/cpt.2212. Epub 1 May 2021. PMID: 33615448; PMCID: PMC8518426.

32. Greenhalgh T., Howick J., Maskrey N. 'Evidence based medicine: a movement in crisis?' *BMJ*, 13 June 2014;348:g3725. doi:10.1136/bmj.g3725.

33. Downs J. *Maladies of Empire: How Colonialism, Slavery, and War Transformed Medicine*. Cambridge, MA: The Bellknap Press of Harvard University Press, 2021.

34. Foucault M. *The Birth of the Clinic: An Archaeology of Medical Perception*. London: Vintage Books, 1994.

35. Kidd I.J., Carel H. 'Healthcare Practice, Epistemic Injustice, and Naturalism'. In Barker S. *et al.* (eds.). *Harms and Wrongs in Epistemic Practice*. Cambridge: Cambridge University Press, 2018. PMID: 32997467.

36. McGill Qualitative Health Research Group. @MQHRG. Twitter.com, 30 September 2015. https://twitter.com/mqhrg/status/649297142859857920?s=20 [accessed 20 February 2024].

37. Greenhalgh T., Annandale E., Ashcroft R. *et al.* 'An open letter to the BMJ editors on qualitative research' [published correction appears in *BMJ*, 2016;352:i957]. *BMJ*, 2016;352:i563. Published 10 February 2016. doi:10.1136/bmj.i563.

38. Loder E., Groves T., Schroter S., Merino J.G., Weber W. 'Qualitative research and The BMJ'. *BMJ*, 2016;352:i641. Published 10 February 2016. doi:10.1136/bmj.i641.

39. Kai J. 'What worries parents when their preschool children are acutely ill, and why: a qualitative study'. *BMJ*, 19 October 1996;313(7063):983-6. doi: 10.1136/bmj.313.7063.983. PMID: 8892420; PMCID: PMC2352339.

40. Reiss J. and Sprenger J. 'Scientific Objectivity'. In Zalta E.N. (ed.). *The Stanford Encyclopedia of Philosophy* (Winter 2020 Edition). https://plato.stanford.edu/archives/win2020/entries/scientific-objectivity/ [accessed 20 February 2024].

41. Paton M., Naidu T., Wyatt T.R., Oni O., Lorello G.R., Najeeb U., Feilchenfeld Z., Waterman S.J., Whitehead C.R., Kuper A. 'Dismantling the master's house: new ways of knowing for equity and social justice in health professions education'. *Adv Health Sci Educ Theory Pract*, December 2020;25(5):1107-1126. doi: 10.1007/s10459-020-10006-x. Epub 2 November 2020. PMID: 33136279; PMCID: PMC7605342.

42. Seth A. 'The big idea: do we all experience the world in the same way?'. *The Guardian*, 3 October 2022. https://www.theguardian.com/books/2022/oct/03/the-big-idea-do-we-all-experience-the-world-in-the-same-way [accessed 20 February 2024].

43. Noble D.F. *A World Without Women; The Christian Clerical Culture of Western Science*. New York: Knopf, 1992.

44. Traweek S. *Beamtimes and Lifetimes: The World of High Energy Physicists*. Cambridge, MA: Harvard University Press, 1988.

45. Woolf V. *Three Guineas*. London: Hogarth Press, 1938.

46. Krieger N. 'Public Health, Embodied History, and Social Justice: Looking Forward'. *Int J Health Serv*, 2015;45(4):587-600. doi: 10.1177/0020731415595549. Epub 2015 Jul 15. PMID: 26182941.

47. Lombarts K.M.J., Verghese A. 'Medicine Is Not Gender-Neutral – She Is Male'. *N Engl J Med*, 31 March 2022;386(13):1284-1287. doi: 10.1056/NEJMms2116556. PMID: 35353969.

48. Harding S. *Objectivity and Diversity: Another Logic of Scientific Research*. Chicago: University of Chicago Press, 2015.

49. Gross R.E. *Vagina Obscura: An Anatomical Voyage*. New York: WW Norton and Co, 2022.

50. Dhairyawan R., Shah A., Bailey J., Mohammed H. 'Factors associated with bacterial sexually transmitted infections among people of South Asian ethnicity in England'. *Sex Transm Infect*, 6 November 2023:sextrans-2023-055879. doi: 10.1136/sextrans-2023-055879. PMID: 37932032.

51. Feinberg M. 'The Myth of Objective Data'. The MIT Press Reader, 17 April 2023. https://thereader.mitpress.mit.edu/the-myth-of-objective-data/ [accessed 20 February 2024].

52. Feinberg M. *Everyday Adventures with Unruly Data*. Boston, MA: MIT Press, 2022.

53. Price A., Albarqouni L., Kirkpatrick J., Clarke M., Liew S.M., Roberts N., Burls A. 'Patient and public involvement in the design of clinical trials: An overview of systematic reviews'. *J Eval Clin Pract*, February 2018;24(1):240-253. doi: 10.1111/jep.12805. Epub 27 October 2017. PMID: 29076631.

54. Laidlaw L., Hollick R.J. 'Values and value in patient and public involvement: moving beyond methods'. *Future Healthc J*, November 2022, 9 (3) 238-242; doi: 10.7861/fhj.2022-0108.

55. Co-Production Collective. 'What is the value of co-production?'. 27 October 2022. https://www.coproductioncollective.co.uk/news/what-is-the-value-of-co-production [accessed 20 February 2024].

56. Burgess R.A., Shittu F., Iuliano A. *et al.* 'Whose knowledge counts? Involving communities in intervention and trial design using community conversations'. *Trials*, 2023; 24, 385. https://doi.org/10.1186/s13063-023-07320-1.

57. Bulbeck H. 'About Priority Setting Partnerships'. James Lind Alliance, 2024. https://www.jla.nihr.ac.uk/about-the-james-lind-alliance/about-psps.htm [accessed 20 February 2024].

58. Partridge N., Scadding J. 'The James Lind Alliance: patients and clinicians should jointly identify their priorities for clinical trials'. *The Lancet*, 27 November–3 December 2004;364(9449):1923-4. doi: 10.1016/S0140-6736(04)17494-1. PMID: 15566996.

59. Chicago Beyond. 'Why am I always being researched?' https://chicagobeyond.org/researchequity/ [accessed 20 February 2024].

6: Roar

1. Nataloff. 'Vito Russo "Why We Fight" speech (corrected video)'. YouTube, 8 November 2015. https://www.youtube.com/watch?v=CoQ8poHCQEs&ab_channel=Nataloff [accessed 20 February 2024].

2. Russo V. 'Why We Fight'. ACT UP demonstration in Albany, New York, 9 May 1988. https://actupny.org/documents/whfight.html [accessed 20 February 2024].

3. ACT UP. 'Home'. https://actupny.com/ [accessed 20 February 2024].

4. Shilts R. *And the Band Played On: Politics, People, and the AIDS Epidemic.* New York: St. Martin's Press, 1987.

5. Buckley Jr. W.R. 'Crucial Steps in Combating the AIDS Epidemic: Identify All the Carriers'. *The New York Times*, 18 March 1986.

6. Ibid.

7. France D. *How to Survive a Plague: The Inside Story of How Citizens and Science Tamed AIDS.* London: Picador, 2016.

8. Hubbard J. (dir.). *United in Anger: A History of ACT UP* documentary film, 6 June 2012.

9. France D. (n 7).

10. Schulman S. *Let the Record Show: A Political History of ACT UP New York, 1987–1993.* New York: Farrar, Straus & Giroux, 2021.

11. Ibid.

12. Concorde Coordinating Committee. 'Concorde: MRC/ANRS randomised double-blind controlled trial of immediate and deferred zidovudine in symptom-free HIV infection.' *The Lancet*, 9 April 1994;343(8902):871-81. PMID: 7908356.

13. Epstein S. *Impure Science: AIDS, Activism and the Politics of Knowledge.* Berkeley, CA: University of California Press, 1998.

14. Palella Jr. F.J., Delaney K.M., Moorman A.C. *et al.* 'Declining morbidity and mortality among patients with advanced human immunodeficiency virus infection'. HIV Outpatient Study Investigators. *N Engl J Med*, 1998;338(13):853-860. doi:10.1056/NEJM199803263381301.

15. Gray D.M. (dir.). *Fire in the Blood* documentary film, 23 January 2013. Available at Dharma Documentaries. 'Fire in the Blood'. YouTube, 20 December 2020. https://www.youtube.com/watch?v=uMsseS_Lqso&ab_channel=DharmaDocumentaries.

16. Gray D.M. (dir.). *Fire in the Blood* transcript. Media Education Foundation, 2013. https://www.mediaed.org/transcripts/Fire-In-The-Blood-Transcript.pdf [accessed 20 February 2024].

17. Eban K. 'How an Indian tycoon fought Big Pharma to sell AIDS drugs for $1 a day'. Quartz, 15 July 2019. https://qz.com/india/1666032/how-indian-pharma-giant-cipla-made-aids-drugs-affordable [accessed 20 February 2024].

18. KFF. 'The U.S. President's Emergency Plan for AIDS Relief (PEPFAR)'. 26 July 2023. https://www.kff.org/global-health-policy/fact-sheet/the-u-s-presidents-emergency-plan-for-aids-relief-pepfar/ [accessed 20 February 2024].

19. HIV i-base. 'African advocacy groups call for dismissal of USAID director Natsios after "racist comments"'. 30 July 2001. https://i-base.info/htb/4691 [accessed 20 February 2024].

20. Committee on International Relations. The United States' War on AIDS: Hearing before the Committee on International Relations, US House of Representatives, 107th Congress, 1st session, 7 June 2001. http://commdocs. house.gov/committees/intlrel/hfa72978.000/hfa72978_0.HTM [accessed 20 February 2024].

21. 'Official offers apology'. *The Globe and Mail*, 27 June 2001. https://www. theglobeandmail.com/amp/news/world/official-offers-apology/article4150034/ [accessed 20 February 2024].

22. Mills E.J., Nachega J.B., Buchan I. *et al.* 'Adherence to antiretroviral therapy in sub-Saharan Africa and North America: a meta-analysis'. *JAMA*, 2006;296(6):679-690. doi:10.1001/jama.296.6.679.

23. Attaran A. 'Adherence to HAART: Africans take medicines more faithfully than North Americans'. *PLoS Med*, February 2007;4(2):e83. doi: 10.1371/journal.pmed.0040083. PMID: 17326715; PMCID: PMC1808103.

24. Treatment Action Campaign. 'Our History – Timeline'. https://www.tac.org. za/our-history/ [accessed 20 February 2024].

25. Dubula V. 'A Decade of Fighting for our Lives'. United Nations, *UN Chronicle*. https://www.un.org/en/chronicle/article/decade-fighting-our-lives [accessed 20 February 2024].

26. Meldrum A. 'South African government ends AIDS denial'. *The Guardian*, 28 October 2006. https://www.theguardian.com/world/2006/oct/28/southafrica. aids [accessed 20 February 2024].

27. Chigwedere P., Seage G.R. 3rd, Gruskin S., Lee T.H., Essex M. 'Estimating the lost benefits of antiretroviral drug use in South Africa'. *J Acquir Immune Defic Syndr*, 1 December 2008;49(4):410-5. doi: 10.1097/qai.0b013e31818a6cd5. PMID: 19186354.

28. Dubula V. 'Our struggle is not over: Vuyiseka Dubula at TEDxEuston'. TEDx Talks, YouTube, 28 January 2014. https://www.youtube.com/watch?v=T2gEbUcFle4&ab_channel=TEDxTalks [accessed 20 February 2024].

29. UNAIDS. 'Global AIDS Strategy 2021-2026 – End Inequalities. End AIDS.' 25 March 2021. https://www.unaids.org/en/resources/documents/2021/2021-2026-global-AIDS-strategy [accessed 20 February 2024].

30. UNAIDS. 'Global HIV & AIDS statistics – Fact sheet'. 2023. https://www. unaids.org/en/resources/fact-sheet [accessed 20 February 2024].

31. Epstein S. (n 13).

32. Reid M.J.A., Arinaminpathy N., Bloom A. *et al.* 'Building a tuberculosis-free world: The Lancet Commission on tuberculosis'. *The Lancet*, 2019; 393(10178):1331-1384. doi:10.1016/S0140-6736(19)30024-8.

33. Nous Group. 'Independent review to address discrimination and advance anti-racism'. London School of Hygiene and Tropical Medicine, 8 December 2021. https://www.lshtm.ac.uk/media/56316 [accessed 20 February 2024].

34. Daftary A., Frick M., Venkatesan N. *et al.* 'Fighting TB stigma: we need to apply lessons learnt from HIV activism'. *BMJ Global Health*, 2017;2:e000515. https://doi.org/10.1136/bmjgh-2017-000515.

35. Zarocostas J. 'Nandita Venkatesan: a voice of hope for tuberculosis survivors'. *The Lancet*, 2019;393(10178):1277. doi:10.1016/S0140-6736(19)30582-3.

36. Terrence Higgins Trust. 'How it all began'. https://www.tht.org.uk/our-work/about-our-charity/our-history/how-it-all-began [accessed 20 February 2024].

37. Smith S. *A Positive Life: HIV from Terrence Higgins to Today* podcast. BBC Sounds, 2022. Available on https://www.bbc.co.uk/sounds/brand/pocgd4vm.

38. aidsmap. 'Who We Are'. https://www.aidsmap.com/about-us/who-we-are [accessed 20 February 2024].

39. *The Mail on Sunday*. 'Britain Threatened by Gay Virus Plague'. *The Mail on Sunday*, 6 January 1985.

40. Glass D. *Queer Footprints: A Guide to Uncovering London's Fierce History*. London: Pluto Press, 2023.

41. Bodies Are Telling. *Body and Soul: We Were Always Here* podcast. Apple Podcasts, Broccoli Productions, 2023–2024. Available at: https://podcasts.apple.com/gb/podcast/body-and-soul-we-were-always-here/id1587035513?i=1000541299849.

42. Mendel G. 'The Ward'. 2024. https://gideonmendel.com/the-ward/ [accessed 20 February 2024].

43. Namiba A., Nyirenda C., Sachikonye M., Mbewe R., Ssanyu Sseruma W. *Our Stories Told by Us: Celebrating the African Contribution to the UK HIV Response*. London: ZZUK Press, 2023.

44. HIV i-base. 'About us'. 2024. https://i-base.info/about-us/ [accessed 20 February 2024].

45. Namiba A. *et al.* (n 43).

46. Shah P.N., Iatrakis G.M., Smith J.R., Wells C., Barton S.E., Kitchen V.S., Kourounis G., Steer P.J. 'Women with HIV presenting at three London clinics between 1985–1992'. *Genitourin Med*, December 1993;69(6):439-40. doi: 10.1136/sti.69.6.439. PMID: 8282296; PMCID: PMC1195147.

47. Shepherd J. ' "We can't be perfect all the time": Life with HIV before anti-retrovirals: A narrative analysis of early published stories by women with HIV in the United Kingdom'. *Women's Health*, 2022;18. doi:10.1177/17455057221078726.

48. Sophia Forum and The Terrence Higgins Trust. 'HIV and Women: Invisible

No Longer – A Call to Action'. April 2018. https://sophiaforum.net/index.php/hiv-and-women-invisible-no-longer/ [accessed 20 February 2024].

49. Petretti S. 'Saluting the Women Who Created Positively Women'. *Positively UK*, 7 March 2022. https://positivelyuk.org/2022/03/07/international-womens-day-saluting-the-women-who-created-positively-women/ [accessed 20 February 2024].

50. O'Sullivan S., Thomson K., Gilchrist S. (eds.) *Positively Women: Living with AIDS*. London: Sheba Feminist Press, 1992.

51. Roche J. ' "It's A Sin" is beautiful, but it neglects the women who also died of AIDS'. *i News*, 29 January 2021. https://inews.co.uk/opinion/its-a-sin-is-beautiful-but-it-neglects-the-women-who-also-died-of-aids-848579 [accessed 20 February 2024].

52. Sophia Forum and The Terrence Higgins Trust. (n 48).

53. Sophia Forum. 'We Are Still Here'. 2019. https://sophiaforum.net/index.php/we-are-still-here/ [accessed 20 February 2024].

54. Stutterheim S.E., van Dijk M., Wang H., Jonas K.J. 'The worldwide burden of HIV in transgender individuals: An updated systematic review and meta-analysis'. *PLoS ONE*, 16(12):e0260063. 2021. https://doi.org/10.1371/journal.pone.0260063.

55. The People First Charter. 'About Us'. https://peoplefirstcharter.org/ [accessed 20 February 2024].

56. Positively UK. 'National Standards for Peer Support in HIV'. HIV Peer Support, 2024. https://hivpeersupport.com/ [accessed 20 February 2024].

57. Ndebele N. 'Hearing is believing: the talking books sharing HIV information in South Africa – a photo essay'. *The Guardian*, 27 December 2022. https://amp.theguardian.com/global-development/2022/dec/27/talking-books-sharing-hiv-information-in-south-africa [accessed 20 February 2024].

58. Modern Art for South Africa. 'Welcome'. https://modernartforsouthafrica.co.za [accessed 20 February 2024].

59. Definition of 'patient' in *Oxford English Dictionary*. https://www.oed.com/dictionary/patient_adj [accessed 20 February 2024].

60. Hanley A., Meyer J. *Patient Voices in Britain, 1840–1948*. Manchester: Manchester University Press, 2021.

61. The Patients Association. 'A brief history of the Patients Association'. 24 April 2023. https://www.patients-association.org.uk/a-brief-history-of-patients-association [accessed 20 February 2024].

62. International Alliance of Patients' Organizations. 'History'. https://www.iapo.org.uk/history [accessed 20 February 2024].

63. World Patients Alliance. 'Who We Are'. 2021. https://www.worldpatientsalliance.org/who-we-are/ [accessed 20 February 2024].

64. Wehling P., Viehöver W., Koenen S. *The Public Shaping of Medical Research:*

Patient Associations, Health Movements and Biomedicine. Oxfordshire: Routledge, 2014.

65. Gilbert D. *The Patient Revolution: How We Can Heal the Healthcare System*. London: Jessica Kingsley Publishers, 2019.

7: Justice

1. Issa H. 'The Unsung'. Literature Wales, 4 July 2023. https://www.literature-wales.org/lw-news/national-poet-of-wales-marks-75th-anniversary-of-the-nhs/ [accessed 20 February 2024].

2. Manthorpe J., Iliffe S., Gillen P., Moriarty J., Mallett J., Schroder H., Currie D., Ravalier J., McFadden P. 'Clapping for carers in the Covid-19 crisis: Carers' reflections in a UK survey'. *Health Soc Care Community*, July 2022;30(4):1442-1449. doi: 10.1111/hsc.13474. Epub 14 June 2021. PMID: 34125450; PMCID: PMC8444820.

3. Howard S. 'Beefed up security or blocking patients: how to respond to patient violence'. *BMJ*, 10 May 2023;381:p995. https://doi.org/10.1136/bmj.p995.

4. Campbell D. 'Satisfaction with the NHS plummets to lowest level in 40 years'. *The Guardian*, 29 March 2023. https://www.theguardian.com/society/2023/mar/29/satisfaction-with-the-nhs-plummets-to-lowest-level-in-40-years [accessed 20 February 2024].

5. Campbell D. 'NHS vacancies in England at "staggering" new high as almost 10% of posts empty'. *The Guardian*, 1 September 2022. https://www.theguardian.com/society/2022/sep/01/nhs-vacancies-in-england-at-staggering-new-high-as-almost-10-of-posts-empty [accessed 20 February 2024].

6. Dhairyawan R., Chetty D. 'Avoiding the Blame Game: Reframing Conversations on Racialised Health Inequalities'. Cost of Living Blog, 3 March 2021. https://www.cost-ofliving.net/avoiding-the-blame-game-reframing-conversations-on-racialised-health-inequalities/ [accessed 20 February 2024].

7. Ahmed S. 'Feeling Depleted?'. Feministkilljoys.com, 17 November 2013. https://feministkilljoys.com/2013/11/17/feeling-depleted/ [accessed 20 February 2024].

8. Burke T. and Brown B. 'Tarana Burke and Brené on Being Heard and Seen'. *Unlocking Us with Brené Brown* podcast, March 2020. Available at: https://open.spotify.com/episode/1zLUgXuBxyJJW6s87oZuKt.

9. Giles C. in Gilbert D., *The Patient Revolution: How We Can Heal the Healthcare System*. London: Jessica Kingsley Publishers, 2019.

10. Ahmed S. (n 7).

11. Blackstock U. 'Why Black doctors like me are leaving faculty positions in academic medical centers'. Stat News, 16 January 2020. https://www.statnews.com/2020/01/16/black-doctors-leaving-faculty-positions-academic-medical-centers/ [accessed 16 February 2024].

12. Mitra Kalita S. 'Looking Back on Three Years of Performative Diversity Efforts'. *Charter* in partnership with *TIME*, 27 June 2023. https://time.com/charter/6290473/undoing-workplace-diversity-gains/ [accessed 16 February 2024].

13. Berenstain N. 'Epistemic exploitation'. *Ergo: An Open Access Journal of Philosophy*, 2016, 3, 569–590. doi:10.3998/ergo.12405314.0003.022.

14. Ferner A., Chetty D. *How to Disagree: Negotiate Difference in a Divided World.* London: Aurum Press, 2019.

15. Morrison T. from Portland State University's Oregon Public Speakers Collection: 'Black Studies Center public dialogue. Pt. 2', 30 May 1975 (http://bit.ly/1vO2hLP). Part of the Public Dialogue on the American Dream Theme, via Portland State University Library (http://bit.ly/1q8HG3h). Morrison's speech is entitled 'A Humanist View'. Available from Hereford S. The Sistah Girl Next Door: https://shareehereford.com/black-literature/toni-morrison-at-portland-state-1975-nobody-really-thought-that-black-people-were-inferior-full-audio/.

16. Dotson K. 'Conceptualizing Epistemic Oppression'. *Social Epistemology*, 2014;28(2):115–138. doi: 10.1080/02691728.2013.782585.

17. Ferner A., Chetty D. (n 14).

18. Alcoff L.M. 'The Problem of Speaking for Others'. *Cultural Critique*, No. 20 (Winter, 1991–1992), pp5–32. University of Minnesota Press: http://www.jstor.org/stable/1354221.

19. Táíwò O.O. *Elite Capture: How the Powerful Took Over Identity Politics (and Everything Else).* London: Pluto Press, 2022.

20. @DrBlackDeer. Twitter.com, 28 May 2023. https://twitter.com/drblackdeer/status/1662956413746806785 [accessed 20 February 2024].

21. Ahmed S. 'Making Feminist Points'. Feministkilljoys.com, 11 September 2013. https://feministkilljoys.com/2013/09/11/making-feminist-points/?amp [accessed 20 February 2024].

22. Lorde A. 'The Transformation of Silence Into Language and Action' in *The Cancer Journals.* London: Penguin Random House, 2020.

23. Lorde A. *A Burst of Light: Living with Cancer.* Michigan: Firebrand Books, 1988.

Conclusion

1. Manne K. *Down Girl: The Logic of Misogyny.* London: Penguin Books, 2019.

2. Roberts L. 'NHS spends more than £8.2m on "woke warriors" in diversity jobs'. *The Telegraph*, 26 December 2022. https://www.telegraph.co.uk/news/2022/12/26/nhs-spends-82m-woke-warriors-diversity-jobs/ [accessed 20 February 2024].

3. Leary A. 'Lessons Not Learned' *BMJ*, 2023; 382:p1943. https://doi.org/10.1136/bmj.p1943.

4. Francis G. *Free for All: Why the NHS Is Worth Saving.* London: Profile Books, 2023.

5. General Medical Council. 'The state of medical education and practice in the UK: workplace experiences 2023'. https://www.gmc-uk.org/about/what-we-do-and-why/data-and-research/the-state-of-medical-education-and-practice-in-the-uk#foreword [accessed 20 February 2024].

6. Marmot M., Allen J., Boyce T. *et al.* 'Health Equity in England: The Marmot Review 10 Years On'. London: Institute of Health Equity, 2010.

7. Positive East. 'PE Home'. https://www.positiveeast.org.uk/ [accessed 20 February 2024].

8. The Terrence Higgins Trust. 'Home'. https://www.tht.org.uk/ [accessed 20 February 2024].

9. The Food Chain. 'Home'. https://www.foodchain.org.uk/ [accessed 20 February 2024].

10. World Health Organization. 'Refugee and migrant health'. 2 May 2022. https://www.who.int/news-room/fact-sheets/detail/refugee-and-migrant-health [accessed 20 February 2024].

11. 'Anti-LGBT laws continue to hinder the HIV response'. *The Lancet HIV*, 2022, 9(10). https://doi.org/10.1016/S2352-3018(22)00265-X.

12. Coen-Sanchez K., Ebenso B., El-Mowafi I.M. *et al.* 'Repercussions of overturning Roe v. Wade for women across systems and beyond borders'. *Reprod Health*, 2022 (19, 184). https://doi.org/10.1186/s12978-022-01490-y.

13. Bawden A. 'Martha's rule: what it will mean for patients and their families'. *The Guardian*, 14 September 2023. https://amp.theguardian.com/politics/2023/sep/14/marthas-rule-what-it-will-mean-for-patients-and-their-families [accessed 20 February 2024].

14. Wong C. 'UK first to approve CRISPR treatment for diseases: what you need to know'. *Nature*, 16 November 2023. https://www.nature.com/articles/d41586-023-03590-6 [accessed 20 February 2024].

15. Royal College of Obstetricians and Gynaecologists. 'Menopause and later life'. https://www.rcog.org.uk/for-the-public/menopause-and-later-life/ [accessed 20 February 2024].

16. Ahmed K. 'Cost of tuberculosis treatment halved in deal to permit generic versions'. *The Guardian*, 31 August 2023. https://amp.theguardian.com/global-development/2023/aug/31/cost-of-tuberculosis-treatment-halved-in-deal-to-permit-generic-versions [accessed 20 February 2024].

17. Peralta F. and Healing Justice London. 'What is health justice?'. *Shado*, 9 August 2023. https://shado-mag.com/know/what-is-health-justice/ [accessed 20 February 2024].

18. Ibid.

19. Patel R. and Marya R. *Inflamed: Deep Medicine and the Anatomy of Injustice.* London: Allen Lane, 2021.

20. Mulcahy E. 'Doing the right thing for a kinder, fairer, and greener health and care service'. *BMJ*, 2023;382:p1905. doi: 10.1136/bmj.p1905.

21. Farmer P. quoted by Partners in Health. '5 Quotes from Paul Farmer That Inspire Us'. 7 April 2022. https://www.pih.org/article/5-quotes-paul-farmer-inspire-us [accessed 20 February 2024].

Acknowledgements

This book is a product of two decades of clinical practice and so my biggest thanks go to the patients, colleagues and advocates I've met in that time. You've taught me how to be a better doctor and I continue to try to improve every day. I'm grateful to my NHS and academic colleagues who kindly gifted me the time and space I needed to concentrate on writing. Thank you to the community organisations advancing health justice and amplifying minoritised voices that I've had the honour of collaborating with. These include 4M Mentor Mothers, NAZ Project, Positively UK, Sophia Forum, Positive East, aidsmap, The Love Tank, Race and Health, Decolonising Contraception/Reproductive Justice Initiative, National AIDS Trust and SAHAR, but there are also many others who have inspired me.

Authoring a book has been a lifelong dream, but writing professionally has been a relatively recent path. I'm grateful to the editors who have encouraged me: Samantha Asumadu at Media Diversified for publishing my first piece on health inequalities; Joanna Palmer at *The Lancet* for treating me like a real writer and giving me the confidence to carry on; and Aoife Molloy at *BMJ Leader* for making me feel like what I had to say was important.

The seeds of this book come from my professional and personal experiences, but they were sown and nurtured by the inaugural Wellcome Collection x Spread the Word scheme for under-represented authors in 2022. This developed my unformed mass of ideas into a credible book proposal, and demystified the publishing process. Thanks to Bobby Nayyar, Francesca Barrie, Ellen Johl and everyone who taught on this scheme. In particular, thanks to my writing mentor, Angela Saini, for thoughtful feedback

that significantly shaped the direction of the book. I was fortunate to share this experience with fellow awardees Aimee Cliff, Dylan Brethour, James Zatka-Haas, Mashal Iftikhar and Masud Husain – you are all so talented and I cannot wait to see your books on shelves!

This book wouldn't exist without the efforts of my wonderful agent Holly Faulks and superb editor Katie Packer. Thank you for believing in the book, and me! I'm also really grateful to the rest of the team at Trapeze including Serena Arthur, Susie Bertinshaw, Ilona Jasiewicz and Leanne Oliver. *Unheard*'s striking cover is due to Dan Mogford.

Thank you to Hanan Issa for writing such beautiful poetry and giving me permission to include a section in Chapter 7.

Heartfelt thanks to my interviewees for taking the time to meet me and for their insightful comments. Simon Collins, Giskin Day, Eli Fitzgerald, Riya George, Enam Haque, Jo Josh, Lynn Laidlaw, Shomari Lewis-Wilson, Mala Rao, Winnie Ssanyu Sseruma, Rebecca Tayler Edwards and Jonathon Tomlinson, in your different ways, you are driving change that improves people's health. For conversations about the book's content, invaluable advice on the writing process and for early reading, thank you to Ashlesha Patel, Darren Chetty, Annabel Sowemimo, Anne Hanley, Charlie Hughes, Gita Ralleigh, Madhu Pai, Angelina Namiba, Rebecca Mbewe, Shema Tariq and the Neuwriters.

For general cheerleading and motivation, thank you to my amazing friends, especially Katherine Bellenie, Madeleine Bradnam, Dolly Kapoor, Amy Silberzahn, Michelle Woolfenden, Clare Morden, Amrita Kumar, Caroline Chau and Roxanne Foster.

I'm thankful to my family who have gotten me to this stage. I want to recognise the long line of strong and loving women I come from, especially Mumma, Aai and Mavshi. Thanks to my parents who instilled in me their ethos of hard work, public service and living life to the fullest. I also appreciate their care when I stayed over to write chunks of the book in my childhood bedroom. I'm particularly grateful to my mother for taking me to our neighbour-hood library every weekend for as long as I can remember, ensuring that books would always be a fundamental part of my life. To my sister – I will never grow out of wanting to be a part of Star Club with you.

And lastly, thank you to Darren, my biggest support and partner in everything. In the words of Jarvis Cocker, when I met you 'something changed'.